D0931742

YOU CAN LOOK

Younger

AT ANY AGE

Also by Nelson Lee Novick, M.D.

Saving Face
Skin Care for Teens
Super Skin
Baby Skin
You Can Do Something
About Your Allergies

You Can Look
Younger
AT ANY AGE

A Leading Dermatologist's Guide

Nelson Lee Novick, M.D.

HENRY HOLT AND COMPANY
NEW YORK

Henry Holt and Company, Inc.
Publishers since 1866
115 West 18th Street
New York, New York 10011

Henry Holt® is a registered
trademark of Henry Holt and Company, Inc.

Published in Canada by Fitzhenry & Whiteside Ltd.,
195 Allstate Parkway, Markham, Ontario L3R 4T8.

Library of Congress Cataloging-in-Publication Data
Novick, Nelson Lee.
You can look younger at any age: a leading dermatologist's guide /
Nelson Lee Novick.
p.   cm.
Includes index.
1. Skin—Care and hygiene. 2. Skin—Aging. I. Title.
RL87.N697   1996   95-24962
646.7'26—dc20   CIP
ISBN 0-8050-3971-6

Henry Holt books are available for special
promotions and premiums. For details contact:
Director, Special Markets.

First Owl Book edition—1996

Designed by Paula R. Szafranski

Printed in the United States of America
All first editions are printed on acid-free paper. ∞
1   3   5   7   9   10   8   6   4   2

To my dearest wife and best friend, Meryl,

for all her caring and support.

And to my five sons, Yoni, Yoel, Ariel, Donny, and Avi,

who give my life a special meaning.

Acknowledgments

Special thanks to my office manager, Barbara Jerabek, for her invaluable suggestions and criticism and for the many hours she devoted to proofing the final manuscript.

Contents

Introduction: What This Book Can Do for You

In the Orient, especially in times past, aging members of society were traditionally venerated for their wisdom and experience. But in our culture, there has long been a stigma associated with growing older. Older-appearing persons are typically considered less attractive and are often characterized by such unflattering terms as "wrinkled," "worn-out," and "faded." Studies conducted at Emory University demonstrated that, by contrast, those who "age gracefully" and maintain attractiveness continue to be described in terms suggesting youthfulness, such as having good complexions, smooth skin, and unwrinkled faces. For better or for worse, to be considered attractive in our culture means to look younger.

But good looks and a youthful appearance don't only have a profound effect on the eyes of the beholders. There are important psychological benefits to looking younger and more attractive, such as enhanced self-esteem, which in turn promotes greater self-confidence, better social and professional performance, and greater peer recognition.

Unfortunately, the reverse is often true. In today's youth-oriented culture, the anxiety of aging and the resulting negative perceptions about appearance can initiate a chain reaction beginning with self-doubt and leading to less self-confidence, depression, and finally, withdrawal.

Physical attractiveness can also affect general health and longevity. Recent research at the University of Pennsylvania in the study of older women showed that those who were considered physically attractive registered greater satisfaction with their lives, were more outgoing, more realistic, perceived themselves as having less sickness, and indeed were in better health. In a study of one thousand men, researchers found that those who looked old for their age were, in fact, older in terms of the physiologic functioning of such vital organs as the heart, lungs, and kidneys, and that they were generally less healthy than those who looked younger than their years.

Since it is our skin that exhibits the most visible effects of aging, men and women in ever increasing numbers are seeking ways to have younger-looking skin. Both Hollywood and Madison Avenue have tried to capitalize on this growing market demand. The airwaves are filled with commercials for cosmetic surgery centers, and beauty and fashion magazines are replete with ads for creams, lotions, or makeup that promises an instant end to everything from wrinkles and brown spots to stretch marks and cellulite. Great advances in cosmetic surgery now offer the consumer a huge menu of treatments, from smoothing wrinkles to sucking out jowl, procedures whose results are for the most part gratifying, but may be costly in terms of money, time lost from work, and discomfort during and after surgery.

The array of offerings to help eager consumers look young is dizzying. Some of the products are good, some useless, and some downright bad. Adding to this confusion is the ever growing number of makeover books by cosmeticians and magazine beauty columnists in bookstores across the country. These books frequently present conflicting advice and are often filled more with personal opinions and anecdotes than with hard facts.

The need, therefore, for an up-to-date, medically based, user-friendly guide to consumers for safely and economically achieving healthier and younger-looking skin is clear. This book focuses not only upon what your cosmetic surgeon can do for you, but on what you can do for yourself. It introduces simple skin-beautifying home regimens and in-office procedures known as the 4 Rs—Renovating, Resurfacing, Removing, and Recontouring. Translating confusing medical jargon into plain English, this guide simplifies the theories and clarifies the procedures, providing useful answers and practical recommendations.

In Part One, "Getting Down to Basics," you learn how to determine your skin's age so that you can choose what is best for your skin. In Part Two, "Renovating," you learn important measures for preventing skin aging and how best to use sunscreens, moisturizers, cleansers, and makeups. In Part Three, "Resurfacing," you are introduced to the new age of the "cosmeceuticals" as part of daily, at-home regimens as well as the latest in-office treatments for skin rejuvenation and wrinkle removal, such as fruit washes and skin buffing. Part Four, "Removing," describes a variety of methods for eliminating unsightly facial scars and explains the most common simple surgeries for a more youthful look. Part Five, "Recontouring," explores the injectable use of filler substances, from collagen to fat, for plumping up scars, wrinkles, and furrows. It also examines what you need to know about liposuction for removing unwanted lumps and creating a sleeker facial look. And, in Part Six, "What Else?" you get a broad look at some of the more exciting topical and surgical treatments for aging skin in store for us soon in our continuing, centuries-old search for Ponce de Leon's fountain of youth.

This book was written in hopes of providing the necessary

background for you to become a more knowledgeable consumer of skin health and beauty care, and more confident to participate in all aspects of your own treatment and recommendations. Throughout, I have mentioned a variety of cosmetics and drugs for various conditions by brand name. These products are ones with which I have had considerable personal experience and have found to be consistently effective. I am not, however, endorsing any product or products or any generic substance. In most cases, the products cited are by no means the only products available for dealing with the conditions discussed, nor does exclusion from my list imply that a particular product is not equally effective. If some products have been found worthless, I clearly say so. I do suggest, however, that you consult your dermatologist or cosmetic surgeon if you have any questions about the value or efficacy of a specific drug or cosmetic. The descriptions and explanations of medical therapies and surgical procedures are addressed to the general concerns of a wide audience. This book is not intended to be a substitute for professional advice. Should you have particular concerns about any form of therapy described herein, you should ask your doctor. Finally, the treatment fees and medication prices quoted throughout the book are given as a range, since they may vary considerably from one part of the country to another and even among physicians and suppliers within a particular location.

PART ONE

Getting Down to Basics

1

Know What You're Starting With: Determining Your Skin's Age

Your skin, the largest organ of your body, measures approximately twenty square feet and weighs, on average, between seven and nine pounds. But we have only recently begun to appreciate how complex its structure and functions are. Although you don't need to learn the intricacies of its anatomy and physiology, the more knowledge you have about your skin, the less likely it is that you will fall prey to advertising fluff and inflated marketing promises for beauty products and skin care regimes. You will be a more discriminating consumer, which can save you a lot of time, money, and dashed hopes. You will also be able to appreciate the reasons for the various skin care recommendations and procedures discussed throughout this book. What follows are some of the basics about your skin, what happens to it as you age, and how to determine your skin's real age.

NORMAL SKIN

Your skin is composed of three primary layers—the epidermis, dermis, and subcutis—each with its essential and unique functions.

The epidermis is the highly cellular, uppermost layer of your skin. No thicker than a page in this book, it is composed of between fifteen and twenty overlapping layers that are constantly undergoing a process of birth, life, and death. As older cells are shed at the skin's surface, new cells are constantly being produced by actively dividing cells at the base of the epidermis.

Melanocytes, the pigment-producing cells of your skin, are in the lowermost layer of the epidermis alongside the actively dividing cells. These highly specialized cells produce melanin, the pigment that is responsible for imparting a brownish color to your skin. Racial variations in skin color are attributable to genetically determined differences in both the amount and distribution of melanin within the skin. More than simply giving you color, melanin protects you by absorbing the sun's damaging ultraviolet rays, which are believed to be responsible for premature skin aging and the development of skin cancers (see chapter 2). A suntan is nothing more than increased melanin production following prolonged exposure to the sun.

The topmost layer of the epidermis consists of a sheet of nonliving cells called the *stratum corneum*, or the horny layer, so named because the cells of this layer become tough when tightly compacted, like an animal horn. In fact, the horns of mammals are made of keratin, the same protein material that makes up this layer. The surface of the horny layer is somewhat acidic and is referred to as the acid mantle, a term you will see often in moisturizer advertisements. Abnormal accumulation of horn cells on the surface of your skin, for any reason, can result in distressing skin roughness, ashiness, or flakiness.

The horny layer serves as your skin's primary physical barrier to the environment. It prevents the penetration of most substances that come in contact with your skin or are applied directly to it. Only substances with a molecular size smaller than the size of water molecules can readily penetrate this amazing epidermal barrier. This is why, contrary to what advertisers would have you believe, your skin cannot "eat up" or "drink up" large molecular substances, such as collagen, elastin, vitamins, or nutrients— ingredients often contained in many of the fanciest, most expensive moisturizers and cosmetics (see chapter 3).

Beneath the epidermis lies the dermis, which is the cellular and largely fibrous and elastic supporting layer of your skin. Because it contains the important fibers collagen and elastin, the dermis is the focus of much advertising by moisturizer manufacturers. Collagen and elastin are the complex proteins responsible for the support and elasticity of the skin and are responsible for your skin's ability to retain its original shape after being stretched or pulled. Both proteins are composed of large complex molecules, which are too large to penetrate the skin; therefore, claims that collagen or elastin in moisturizers can permeate aging skin and replace lost natural protein fibers are unfounded.

The dermis also contains an intricate, fifteen-foot-per-square-inch network of small blood vessels that brings nutrition to the skin, as well as a dense network of twiglike nerve endings that are responsible for the sensations of temperature, pressure, vibration, and pain. The small blood vessels also remove metabolic waste materials, regulate body temperature by constricting or dilating as needed in response to changes in outside temperature, and keep your skin healthy-looking.

The bottommost layer of your skin is the subcutis, or fatty layer, which lies immediately below the dermis and functions both as a cushion for your vital internal organs and a reserve-energy storage site for the body. In most cases, the amount and distribution of fat throughout your body is believed to be genetically determined. What to do about too much fat remains a hot subject: There are more than three hundred diet books on the market today.

Hair follicles, sweat glands, and oil glands are located throughout the dermis and subcutis. The oil glands, also called sebaceous glands, lie to the side of the hair follicules and produce sebum, or natural skin oil, a complex mixture of different fats and waxes. Sebum is the oil you feel on your face on a hot, humid day. It is secreted through a small duct that leads directly from the oil gland into the shaft of the hair follicle and travels upward to the skin's surface alongside the hair shaft. There are three thousand oil glands per square inch of facial skin. Dead cells and other debris within the hair follicles are "washed" to the skin's surface by this process. By coating the skin, sebum locks in your skin's natural moisture (water) content and prevents it from drying out.

WHAT HAPPENS WHEN SKIN AGES

In the past few years, we have discovered that the skin is subjected to several distinct kinds of aging processes. Two that deserve special note are chronological aging, simply your inherited or family tendency to age, and photoaging, also known as ultraviolet light–induced (UV-induced) aging, which is due mostly to sun damage. The accumulated effects of sun damage are now recognized to be far more profound than those attributed to the natural aging process.

CHRONOLOGICAL SKIN AGING

If asked, most of us could easily describe the outward appearance of an aging face: changes in facial shape, increased prominence of the nose and ears, thinning of the lips, recession of the gums and teeth, and loss of hair and skin color. In addition, you might also include wrinkling of the natural action lines of the face; general laxity and inelasticity; sagging and jowling; and severe, often widespread, dryness.

Dermatologic investigators and others interested in the aging process have long sought to understand the precise nature of the structural and functional alterations in the skin that account for these outward changes. While we have learned much in the past decade, we do not have all the answers. The following is a basic summary of what we do know about chronological skin aging.

As the epidermis ages, it tends to produce fewer new cells and to repair damaged cells less quickly and less effectively. Cells in the horny layer lose some of their ability to adhere to one another. Melanocytes become fewer and function less efficiently. Together, these changes cause drier, thinner, and more wrinkled skin. They also mean graying and whitening of the hair and the development of patchy areas of depigmentation, or loss of skin color.

Equally dramatic changes occur within the dermis: Cell numbers decrease, elastin fibers degenerate, the rate of collagen production slows, and existing collagen and elastin fibers become increasingly rigid and inelastic. The dermis also becomes thinner and less capable of retaining its moisture content. These changes cause dryness, wrinkles, and sagging. Additionally, the number of dermal blood vessels decreases and nerve endings become abnormal, leading to altered or reduced sensation. Wound healing is generally compromised, and there is usually a reduced ability to clear foreign materials and fluids from the skin.

The sebaceous glands may also suffer. Although glandular output actually diminishes, contributing to the generalized dryness and roughness that is characteristic of aging skin, some glands may undergo a benign but aesthetically displeasing enlargement known as sebaceous hyperplasia (see chapter 9).

Hair follicles are also affected. Both men and women may also complain of some degree of scalp hair loss, which is often accompanied by a slowing growth rate and thinning caliber of the remaining hairs. In other areas, such as the ears, nose, and eyebrows of men, and the upper lip and chin of women, previously fine, barely perceptible hairs often become thicker and more visible.

Aging also takes its toll on the fat layer. Shrinking of the subcutis occurs particularly in the face, hands, feet, and shins, creating a more bony-looking appearance. Increased amounts of fat are typically redistributed to the waist in men, and the thighs in women, problems that are exacerbated by the natural decline in the basal metabolic rate that comes with aging and the adoption of a more sedentary lifestyle.

PHOTOAGING

Overwhelming medical evidence indicates that your skin can be badly and irreversibly damaged by years of overexposure to the sun, but most people continue to confuse the effects of photoaging with those resulting from chronological aging. While there is little doubt that sun damage contributes to, accelerates, and exaggerates the effects of chronological skin aging, it causes its own distinctive pattern of "aging," which includes the leathery, hidelike appearance of skin on the face, the V of the chest, and the backs of the hands. Sun damage is also capable of promoting the development of a fishnetlike appearance of numerous "broken" blood vessels on the face and neck, as well as discolorations, thickened age spots (called seborrheic keratoses), and liver spots (known as lentigines), which have nothing to do with either liver disease or natural aging but are the result of accumulated sun damage. The sun is also responsible for promoting the development of dry, scaly, reddish precancers of the skin called actinic keratoses, as well as a variety of overt skin cancers.

To compare the effects of natural aging with sun-induced aging, you need only examine your buttocks (or the area immediately surrounding the nipples in women). If natural aging were the only contributor to skin aging, you would not expect to see much difference between sun-exposed and nonexposed areas. However, you will notice that the sun-protected skin of the buttocks is generally less mottled, less dry, less wrinkled, smoother,

and more supple. That we do so often find such striking differences is a convincing argument for sun protection as one of the
best methods for preventing skin aging.

THREE OTHER SKIN AGING FACTORS

No discussion of skin aging would be complete without mention-
ing the contribution of gravity, facial expressions, and sleep lines
to facial skin aging.

The effects of gravity can be profound. We struggle with its
downward tug on our skin every single day, and the face is particularly susceptible to its effects. When we are upright, gravity
pulls down on our collagen, contributing to the downturned
corners of the mouth, the deep marionettelike furrows on the
sides of the chin, the sagging of the upper and lower eyelids, and
the bulging fat pads under the eyes. The "turkey gobbler" neck,
caused by the downward pull on the thin muscles in the neck,
and the down-pointing chin and nose are other gravity-related
problems.

Expression lines are the "etched" lines that result from moving
our muscles to squint, smile, laugh, frown, chew, and purse our
lips. They may be thought of as the "carvings" of our individual
facial body language into the skin. The horizontal lines across the
forehead or the vertical lines around the lips are examples of
expression lines.

Sleep lines result from the position in which we sleep night
after night. By repeatedly sleeping in a particular position, we
crease our skin, much the same way we indelibly crease paper
by folding it. Curiously, men seem to get sleep lines diagonally
across the forehead, while women typically get them on the
cheeks. Taken together, the effects of gravity, expression lines,
and sleep lines may be thought of as wear-and-tear skin aging.

FACING THE DECADES

The rate at which our skin ages is different for each of us. How soon we see certain changes depends upon the interplay of the five factors just discussed. Nevertheless, there is a general time-table of skin aging for most people's faces.

In one's twenties the skin is usually at its optimum: glowing and elastic and actively renewing itself. Toward the late twenties, however, renewal begins to slow down, and a few fine expression lines may appear. Usually, they are visible only when the face is active, such as when smiling or squinting.

In the thirties, typically at about age thirty-five, wrinkles begin appearing on the thin skin of the eyelids and around the mouth, as well as across the forehead. Although the jawline and neckline remain smooth, the upper eyelids gradually grow hooded. Toward the end of this decade, smile lines may make their appearance.

In the forties, the effects of sun damage from as far back as thirty years become apparent. Crow's-feet (squinting) lines appear at the outer corners of the eyes (sometimes accompanied by dark circles and puffiness under them), forehead "worry" lines become more prominent, as do the "scowl" lines between the eyes. Liver spots, mottled discolorations, and keratoses may become evident, and decreasing estrogen (common at this time of life) may con-tribute to thinning skin. The nose may begin to droop slightly from the effects of gravity.

In the fifties, the tip of the nose may point downward, the eye-brows may droop, a double chin may become apparent, sagging and jowling of the skin become more evident, and bags under the eyes appear. In addition, arcs, creases, and grooves continue to deepen, and there is a progressive overall loss of elasticity. As skin sags and repositions itself along the face, prominent features such as high cheekbones, a large nose, or a wide forehead become more apparent.

In the sixties and beyond, facial lines and furrows intensify and curve downward. The skin becomes generally drier, rougher, more leathery, and inelastic and may be covered with age spots. Jowls and a pronounced double chin redrape the face, while the upper eyelids become hooded and drooping and the lower eyelid bags increasingly protrude. At varying rates, the earlobes droop, the nose enlarges and becomes bonier-looking, and the tip of the nose flattens and points farther downward.

While this timetable may sound like a relentless process toward doom and gloom, you should remember that not everyone follows this pattern in the same way or at the same rate. People who are in their twenties who have had loads of sun exposure when they were young children or teenagers may have skin that resembles that of a forty-year-old. Conversely, others in their late forties may have the skin of a twenty-five-year-old, for a combination of reasons.

But perhaps most important, the timetable describes individuals who have allowed nature to take its course, without doing much about it. Happily, these days, few people need resign themselves to the timetable. There are many things that can be done to combat, slow, or even reverse the signs of aging.

HOW YOU'RE DOING—A QUICK DIAGNOSTIC SKIN CHECK

Having learned the general timetable of skin aging, now would be a good time to take stock of just how well your skin has done up to now. The following is a modification of a six-question questionnaire recently developed to help cosmetic dermatology patients to determine whether their apparent skin age matches their actual chronological age. After examining your face and neck using a magnifying hand mirror and in bright light, preferably sunlight, grade each of the following conditions with 0 for not present; 1 for mild; 2 for moderate; and 3 for severe. When you are finished, total your score.

1) Dry, coarse, roughened, or leathery-appearing skin texture rather than smooth, supple, and slightly oily _____
2) Wrinkling around the mouth or crepe-paper-like crinkling under the eyes, particularly with facial movements _____
3) Wrinkling in the "smile," "scowl," "worry," and "lipstick-bleeding" regions _____
4) Lack of firmness in skin and its inability to bounce back quickly when pinched; sagging, drooping, or jowls at the eyelids and corners of the mouth _____
5) Freckling, mottled and uneven discolorations, and liver spots _____
6) Visible tiny reddish or purplish blood vessels across the nose and cheeks _____

Total Score: _____

SCORE	AGE
0–2	20–25
3–5	26–35
6–8	36–45
9–11	46–55
12 or higher	56+

If you are disappointed with your score and your skin appears older than you are, take heart. The remainder of this book is for you.

PART TWO

Renovating

2

You Can't Start
Too Soon:
"An Ounce of
Prevention . . ."

If there is one point I would like to emphasize, it is that for most
people, having healthier and younger-looking skin is not a matter
of luck or magic. Instead, it usually requires at least some degree of
commitment and effort. In the last chapter, you learned about what
your skin is made of and what happens to it as you age. In this
chapter, you will learn about the single most crucial aspect of
proper preventive skin maintenance and by far the single best anti-
wrinkle remedy currently available: adequate sun protection. The
effects of diet, exercise, and stress on the skin are also discussed.

THE BARE FACTS

Scientists have long known that, aside from the visible light rays
that we see, the sun emits several different types of harmful invis-
ible radiation, including ultraviolet light A (UVA) and ultraviolet
light B (UVB), which are capable of piercing our atmosphere and

tanning and burning our skin. Scientists have also identified a
third type, called infrared radiation (heat radiation), which may
also be responsible for short- and long-term skin damage.

Despite an intensive public education campaign by many
important organizations, including the American Academy of
Dermatology and the Skin Cancer Foundation, many Americans
today remain "sun worshipers," addicted to tanning and sunbathing. Even less avid devotees of the sun still "ultraviolate" their
skin when they proudly show off that "healthy," golden tan from
their vacation. In a recent study, 51 percent of those polled did
report using a sunscreen last year to minimize the dangers of sun
exposure, but fewer than 40 percent gave "prevention of tanning"
as their reason for doing so. Another study demonstrated that
more than 90 percent of the respondents were aware that sun
exposure is unhealthy, but more than half of them still actively
sought a tan. More than two-thirds of those people studied
admitted to looking better and healthier with a tan, and more
than one out of every ten of them had patronized a tanning salon.
In a sense, sunbathing is like cigarette smoking: Many people
know it's not good, but they can't or won't stop.

THE DARK SIDE OF THE SUN

The following sobering statistics should give even the most dedi-
cated sun lovers pause for thought. At present, scientific evidence
suggests that more than 90 percent of the lifetime medical damage (both precancers of the skin and skin cancers) to your skin is
the result of photoaging, or ultraviolet light–induced skin damage
(see chapter 1). At the same time, sun damage is responsible for
at least 80 percent of all cosmetic damage to your skin (premature aging, wrinkling, sagging, dryness, sallowness, leatheriness,
liver spots, mottling, "broken" blood vessels, and so on). Perhaps
most disturbing is that nearly 80 percent of our lifetime sun damage is completed by the age of eighteen, which is especially

important for parents of children and teenagers to know. When it comes to aging and damaging your skin, the sun is your number-one enemy.

But what about the argument that the sun can also be good for you? Few would deny that a deep tan is attractive or that "catching a few rays" gives many people a psychological uplift. "Sunshine on my shoulders makes me happy," attests a line from one of John Denver's popular songs, pointing to an intimate relationship between people's feelings and the sun. Tanning is also credited with "drying up" colds and pimples and masking acne blemishes, scars, and other types of skin irregularities and discolorations. And doesn't every schoolchild learn that sunlight is crucial for stimulating vitamin D production in our skin, which is necessary for maintaining strong bones and teeth?

The sun possesses no curative power whatsoever. Rather than drying up infections, sun exposure can trigger many cases of herpes virus infections of the lips (cold sores), chicken pox, and warts, as well as some noninfectious conditions. Other people may develop rashes or hives in response to sunlight itself or when exposed to the sun following the use of a particular perfume, cosmetic, soap, detergent, or medication (either applied to the skin or taken internally). And the truth is that all your vitamin D needs can be satisfied in one fifteen-minute daily exposure to the sun. But even this exposure is unnecessary because, with the exception of persons living in underdeveloped countries, most of us get enough vitamin D through the fortified foods we eat, even those people who live on fast-food diets.

Finally, despite the myth, sunlight does not "cure" acne. Actually, most of those who claim that their acne clears up with suntanning find that they break out in whiteheads four to six weeks later. This is probably due to ultraviolet light–induced damage and clogging of the pores beneath the skin's surface. Because of the long gap between cause and effect, most individuals fail to associate their acne flare-up with the sun exposure from several weeks earlier. A tan may be useful for masking blemishes, but there are certainly far safer and more satisfactory ways to accomplish this cosmetically (see chapter 5).

As a dermatologist, I would like to see the Federal Trade Commission (FTC) and Food and Drug Administration (FDA) require that all advertisements for fun-in-the-sun Caribbean and south-of-the-border holidays, as well as any sun products that encourage tanning, to carry the following warning: THE SURGEON GENERAL HAS DETERMINED THAT SUNTANNING IS DANGEROUS TO YOUR HEALTH. SUNTANNING MAY LEAD TO THE DEVELOPMENT OF SKIN CANCERS AND PREMATURE AGING, SAGGING, WRINKLING, AND DISCOLORATION OF THE SKIN.

ON THE BRIGHT SIDE

The good news is that if you like your fun outdoors, you need not hide from the sun. For most of us, complete abstinence from the sun is neither practical nor desirable. Fortunately, safe sun exposure is a matter of knowing your skin type, taking the proper precautions, using the appropriate sunblocking agents and sunscreens, and following a few sensible rules.

Skin Types

Through experience, most of us have a general idea of how sensitive we are to the sun's rays. Some of us always burn and never tan in the sun, and some of us always tan and never burn. Between these two extremes lie a number of individual gradations. Dermatologists refer to these individual differences in sun susceptibility as skin types. Six skin types are currently recognized (see Table 1, page 19). In general, persons with blue eyes and blond hair usually exhibit type I or type II skin; black people are usually type VI. Knowing your skin type is important for selecting the right measures to protect your skin from sunburn and long-term damage.

Table 1 Skin Types

Type I	Always burns; never tans—i.e., extremely sensitive
Type II	Always burns; sometimes tans—i.e., very sensitive
Type III	Sometimes tans; sometimes burns—i.e., sensitive
Type IV	Always tans; sometimes burns—i.e., minimally sensitive
Type V	Always tans; never burns—i.e., not sensitive
Type VI	Negroid skin—always tans (gets darker); sometimes burns—i.e., minimally sensitive

Skin types can generally be grouped along ethnic lines. Persons of Celtic (Scotch-Irish), Scandinavian, or Northern European extraction usually fall into types I or II. Those of Mediterranean backgrounds, such as Italians, Spaniards, and Greeks, are often type III, IV, or V. Asians and Hispanics frequently have type V skin, and sub-Saharan Africans have type VI.

Naturally, individuals within any ethnic or racial grouping may vary in their individual susceptibility to the sun. For example, you might find light-complected blacks having type II or type III skin, or Northern Italians with type I or II. No matter what your ethnic background, it is important to know your specific skin type.

DRESSING FOR OUTDOOR SUCCESS

Choosing the right kinds of protective clothing for outdoor work or play is important. Broad-brimmed hats, wide or wraparound sunglasses, long-sleeved shirts, and long pants offer optimal sun protection. Light-colored, lightweight, tightly woven cotton clothing is best for both comfort and sun protection. While dark clothing is generally more efficient at absorbing the harmful rays, it also absorbs more heat and is less comfortable for warm-weather wear. Loose weaves let too much light through. In addition, wet, clinging clothing can transmit ultraviolet light, so beware if you tend to perspire heavily or if you place dry clothing directly over a wet body at the beach or poolside.

Since cataracts (opacification of the lenses of the eyes) have also been associated with lifelong exposure to ultraviolet rays, your choice of sunglasses is important, too. Select them with more than just fashion in mind. Look for those that block out 99 percent of the ultraviolet light. Recent evidence confirms that ordinary dark glasses do indeed reduce glare, but by cutting down on light and allowing your pupils to dilate, more potentially damaging ultraviolet rays may reach the delicate retinas of your eyes. Polarized lenses that are tinted dark green, dark brown, or gray are good choices, while yellow or rosé-colored sunglasses are less effective and less safe. If you have specific questions on the safest eyewear for you, consult your eye care specialist.

SUNBLOCKS AND SUNSCREENS

Sunblocks and sunscreens are your next line of defense against the sun's rays. While both agents prevent ultraviolet light contact with your skin, they do so in different ways. Sunblocks act as a physical barrier to incoming ultraviolet light and work by reflecting the harmful rays away from your skin. Sunscreens work by directly absorbing harmful ultraviolet radiation from your skin rather than scattering it away.

Sunblocks may be found in ointment, cream, or lotion forms and usually contain either titanium dioxide, zinc oxide, kaolin, or talc. Sunblocks are very effective products, but until recently, they were somewhat limited in their usefulness because of their thickness and greasiness and their tendency to discolor clothing.

For those reasons, they were usually reserved for especially sun-sensitive regions, such as the nose and lips. (A thick white zinc-oxide ointment nose coat was for years the hallmark of the beach lifeguard.) To make their products more aesthetically pleasing, several manufacturers formulated them as beige (RV-Paque and A-Fil creams) or brightly colored preparations (Le-Zink). More recently, manufacturers have been incorporating a new, finely ground (micronized) form of titanium dioxide into their sun-protection and cosmetic products. These sunblocking products, often called chemical-free sunscreens because they do not contain other sunscreen ingredients (see below), are quite effective and do not have the problems associated with the previous versions. Examples of these products include Neutrogena Chemical-Free Sunblocker SPF-17 and Elizabeth Arden Basic Block Non-Chemical Sunscreen SPF-21.

Sunscreens are not considered cosmetics and are classified as drugs by the FDA. PABA and PABA-esters (padimate-O and padimate-A) were the most commonly used sunscreen ingredients; more recently, a wide variety of other effective ingredients have been added to the list, including benzophenones, cinnamates, salicylates, and avobenzone (Parsol 1789, at present the most effective commercially available ingredient for screening UVA radiation). Many scientists now believe that sunscreens can prevent the long-term damaging effects of sun exposure, although this has not been conclusively demonstrated. We do know for sure that, when used appropriately, sunscreens can prevent sunburn and reduce or prevent tanning.

Although the long-term damaging effects of sun exposure were once held to be irreversible, recent investigations indicate otherwise. A study using laboratory animals showed that the regular application of potent sunscreens not only prevented further ultraviolet light–induced damage but allowed sun-damaged skin to repair itself, despite continued exposure. In a recent study of six hundred persons in Australia, investigators found that regular sunscreen application actually reversed precancerous lesions to normal—another powerful argument for the regular use of sunscreens.

By now, the sun protection factor (SPF) labeling on sunscreens and other cosmetics is probably old hat for most of you. As a rule, sunscreens with an SPF of 8 or less provide minimal protection. Those with SPFs between 8 and 15 provide moderate protection. Maximum-protection sunscreens are those with SPF of 15 or higher. This means, for example, if you would normally burn after twenty minutes in the first blush of the spring sun, using a sunscreen with an SPF of 10 would allow you to spend ten times that twenty minutes (or more than three hours) in the sun before reaching that same degree of sunburn under the same conditions.

In general, the fairer and more sensitive your skin, the higher the SPF sunscreen you should choose. Those with type I or II skin should use maximum-protection sunscreens. Those with type III or IV may use sunscreens with an SPF of 8 or higher. Dark-skinned blacks generally need no sunscreens at all.

Sunscreens, particularly those containing PABA or its derivatives, can sometimes cause problems themselves. They occasionally cause stinging when applied to the skin, especially the face. They can stain clothing yellow or yellow-orange and can also cause skin allergies, alone or in combination with sunlight. Even more important, their use on the skin can cause certain individuals to become allergic to such common anesthetics as benzocaine and procaine, to hair dyes containing para-phenylenediamene, and to sulfonamide antibiotics. For intensive outdoor protection, I usually advise my patients to use a maximum-protection, PABA-free, fragrance-free sunscreen, such as Shade UVAGuard. And for everyday use, a dual-purpose, under-makeup moisturizer/sunscreen, such Oil of Olay UV Protectant, would be wise. If you have a tendency toward acne, make certain your sunscreen is also labeled *nonacnegenic* and *noncomedogenic*.

You should routinely—not just when you're going to the beach or out golfing—apply a sunscreen daily between mid-April and mid-October, when the sun is high in the sky and its rays more direct. You can accumulate a lot of long-term damage to your skin just from short walks in the noonday sun between buildings or that ten-minute coffee break in the park. And be sure to use sunscreens when skiing. High altitudes and thin air permit more ultraviolet light–damage, and snow and ice can reflect as much as 90 percent of the sun's rays.

For best results, you should apply your sunscreen fifteen to thirty minutes before going outside, preferably while in a dry, air-conditioned room to allow the sunscreen enough time to bind to your skin. Apply liberally and use a sufficient amount of sunscreen to form a protective film on your skin; do not rub it in. Remember to reapply sunscreen after every two hours of vigorous exercise, since sweat can dilute its benefits. Always reapply immediately after swimming, even if your sunscreen claims to be waterproof. But keep in mind that reapplication does not increase the length of time you can stay out in the sun; it only restores the original SPF potency of the product. The newer sports sunscreens do stay on longer, but they tend to be heavier and may clog pores. Lips are especially sensitive to sun damage; so make certain to protect them with lip balms containing high SPF ingredients (Total Eclipse, Chapstick-15).

Don't confuse sunscreens with suntan products containing mineral oil, mineral oil and iodine, baby oil, cocoa butter, and coconut oil. Unless these lotions also contain active sunscreen ingredients, they do nothing more than lubricate your skin. They may, in fact, make matters worse by acting as a lens, focusing the sun's rays on your skin.

If you still insist on getting a tan, do it prudently. Start with a higher-SPF sunscreen for about two days, then cut back to a lower-SPF sunscreen until you become as dark as you wish. At that point, return to using the higher-SPF product; once you are tan, you will get enough of the UVA through the sunscreen to maintain your tan. Never forget, though: "Today's tan is tomorrow's wrinkle."

OTHER IMPORTANT REMINDERS

Pay attention to those new regional UV index reports usually included with the daily weather forecast on radio, television, or in your local newspaper during the summer months. They give you a good idea of how strong the sun is in your area and how much caution you should exercise. Avoid outdoor exposure during the hours between 10 A.M. and 2 P.M., when the sun is directly overhead. That does not mean, however, that you need not use a sunscreen before or after those hours; sun-induced damage can occur all day long. Take extra care during particularly hot, humid, or windy periods, which are known to enhance the harmful effects of ultraviolet radiation. And because ultraviolet light can penetrate up to three feet of water, you must use sunscreens before swimming as well as after. Be warned that water droplets beaded on your skin can intensify the sun's rays.

Don't let your guard down in shady places or on cloudy days. Use sunscreens even if you intend to sit under the boardwalk, a beach umbrella, or a shade tree. Between 40 and 60 percent of the sun's rays are reflected off the sand, water, and concrete. Cloudy yet bright days can also be quite deceptive. They tend to be cooler and darker, tempting you to stay outdoors longer and use less protection. Nevertheless, ultraviolet rays can pierce clouds and cause a serious sunburn. And never use sun reflectors. They concentrate the sun's harmful rays and focus them on areas ordinarily protected from the sun, such as your eyelids, earlobes, and the underside of your chin.

SUN SENSORS

For those of you who delight in gadgets, you can purchase a new kind of ultraviolet light–sensing device or sun-exposure meter. These pocket-sized devices can be programmed with your skin type and with the SPF of the sunscreen you use and are designed to alert you to possible overexposure. A beep tone sounds when you need to seek shade. A variety of sun-sensing badges—more readily available and considerably less expensive—have also been marketed. Designed to be affixed to your hat or clothing, these badges change colors to alert you when the danger of ultraviolet overexposure is greatest. At present, however, the value and reliability of all sun-sensing devices and badges remains unproven, and I find little to recommend them.

TANNING PARLORS

The appearance of increasing numbers of tanning salons and "sun" centers are another manifestation of the continuing tanning craze. Insofar as tanning salons permit year-round exposure, they are potentially more dangerous than the sun. At present, there are more than ten thousand tanning salons in the United States alone, and approximately two million Americans persist in frequenting them. A typical tanning bed is body-length and surrounds the user with walls of ultraviolet light–radiating fluorescent lights.

Before 1985, tanning salons—having switched in most cases from UVB to UVA—claimed to be "safer than the sun." Since that time, however, it has become illegal for tanning salons to make that claim. While it is true that sunburning is less likely with UVA sources, it is still possible. Other dangers of ultraviolet radiation previously discussed remain quite real. As of September 1986, the FDA requires manufacturers of tanning devices to affix a warning label on all their machines. I echo the FDA concern and strongly caution you against their use. Sunlamps pose a similar danger and likewise should be avoided.

GOOD HEALTH MEANS
HEALTHIER SKIN

Good skin is not merely the result of what you apply to it. The way you live—what you eat, what you drink, what you feel, and whether you exercise—can make big differences in the way you look. After sun exposure, other cardinal sins against both your general health and the health of your skin include improper diet, lack of exercise, unrelenting stress, smoking, alcohol, and drugs.

DIET

Eating a well-balanced diet, which supplies you with enough nutrients for your daily needs plus a surplus of storable nutrients, is the key for staying healthy and avoiding nutrition-related skin problems. To maintain optimal health, you need a diet consisting of plenty of the following nutrients: water, proteins, fats, carbohydrates, vitamins, and minerals. Proteins are needed for cell growth and repair. Carbohydrates provide energy. Fats supply storage energy, and vitamins and minerals are vital assistants for regulating body functioning. And plenty of water is essential for all our metabolic processes.

Since vitamins and minerals have been the subject of so much ad hype, they deserve special mention. Vitamins are organic substances, and minerals are inorganic substances. To date, thirteen vitamins and more than sixteen essential minerals have been identified. The vitamins A, C, D, and E, and the minerals iron, zinc, and calcium are well-known substances that are essential for many aspects of continued good health.

Unquestionably, deficiencies of certain vitamins and minerals can adversely affect your general health and appearance. For example, severe vitamin C deficiency can result in easy bruisability and fragile, bleeding gums; severe deficiencies of vitamin B_6, or niacin, can lead to skin rashes. However, despite what health food stores and vitamin and mineral manufacturers would like you to believe, most people who consume ordinary Western diets, even fast-food junkies, do not usually become vitamin or mineral deficient. Under ordinary circumstances, therefore, most Americans do not need vitamin or mineral supplements.

So far, neither vitamins nor minerals have been proven to possess any magical or curative powers. Taking daily supplements cannot stop you from feeling nervous, help you feel less run-down, make up for a lack of sleep, or cure the common cold. What's more, the vitamin and mineral industry is not well regulated by the government, and there are no guarantees that supplements contain what they say they do or that they break down in your digestive system well enough to be absorbed. On the other hand, it is generally not harmful to take ordinary multivitamin and mineral supplements on a daily basis, so long as you do not exceed the FDA's recommended daily allowances (RDA). One note of caution: Because the mineral iodine can aggravate acne, individuals who are acne-prone should avoid mineral supplements containing iodine. Of course, the best way to get what you need is to eat more fruits and vegetables.

For some time now, there has been a flurry of speculation that certain vitamin and mineral antioxidants, such as beta-carotene, vitamins A, C, and E, and selenium, may be helpful in preventing or reversing UV-induced sun damage. Since there is apparently little risk in overdosing with beta-carotene, vitamin C, and selenium, there is little reason not to supplement your diet with these items if you wish. But this is definitely not the case with vitamin A. While it, too, may have some benefit in preventing sun-induced skin cancers and in healing wounds, there is a substantial risk of serious consequences from overdosing, and it is ill-advised to take it without the advice of a physician.

In addition to the other well-known benefits of a low-fat diet (weight reduction; reduced risks of heart disease, colon cancer, and breast cancer), one more benefit can now be added. Researchers at Baylor College of Medicine in Houston found that people eating a low-fat diet for two years reduced the number of precancerous growths on the skin by about 70 percent as compared to individuals who did not restrict their fat intake. For people who are susceptible to these unsightly, reddish, scaly growths, a change to a low-fat diet would seem reasonable.

EXERCISE

Regular exercise is good both for your general health and for your skin. Working out can improve your skin's color and texture by increasing blood flow, which means the delivery of more oxygen and nutrients to your skin, accounting in large measure for that healthy glow seen after exercise. The increased muscle tone and weight control that frequently result from a regular exercise program further contribute to improving appearance and well-being. Although facial movements can contribute to the formation of expression-line wrinkles, there is no evidence that isometric facial exercises can reverse the etching of the skin once it has occurred.

By taking a few simple precautions to protect your skin while exercising, you can prevent problems and enjoy yourself more. Remove any makeup before beginning your workout to permit better sweat evaporation from the skin. Remove jewelry as well—it may not only get in the way of your workout, but can be responsible for causing allergies and irritation. Costume jewelry, and even gold jewelry, contains some nickel; in nickel-sensitive persons, problems result when small amounts of nickel are leached out of their jewelry by heavy perspiration. If you absolutely will not be seen without jewelry, dust it lightly with some talcum powder to keep the skin areas under it dry, and gently cleanse your skin as soon as possible after working out.

STRESS

It's been written that while the eyes may mirror the soul, the skin can mirror the mind. We know that many skin conditions can be aggravated or triggered by increased nervous tension, including acne, profuse sweating, facial flushing, itching, allergies, eczema, and psoriasis. And as an illustration of the power of mind over matter, warts have been known to disappear suddenly when children have been convinced by their doctors that a placebo wart remedy was really a powerful medication.

The effects of our emotions and stress on our skin is only now beginning to be appreciated. Many doctors have become less reluctant to recommend the use of relaxation and meditation techniques, in addition to the use of conventional medical therapies, for some of their patients with stress-linked skin conditions. Nevertheless, much remains to be learned about our "emotional skin" and how we can best deal with the effect of our emotions.

SMOKING, ALCOHOL, AND DRUGS

Smoking, heavy drinking, or using drugs can wreck your skin and your health in general. The life-threatening consequences of smoking—emphysema, lung cancer, and heart disease—have been well publicized and should be well known to you. However, cigarette smoking can have serious effects on your skin as well. Studies indicate that heavy smokers have sallower, more wrinkled skin than nonsmokers—facial-skin changes referred to as the "smoker's face." Cigarette smoking may also adversely affect wound healing after some forms of surgery. All these problems may be due, at least in part, to the constricting effects of nicotine or other cigarette-smoke byproducts on the skin's small blood vessels. Although publicity about the hazards to the heart and lungs from cigarette smoking has not as yet brought cigarette smoking to a halt, perhaps greater awareness that it can cause severe wrinkling, sagging, and aging of the skin will.

Light drinking, one or two "social drinks" a day, has not been shown to be necessarily unhealthy for the skin. This, of course, does not mean that it is healthy for you, either. Heavy drinking (there are an estimated ten million "problem drinkers" or alcoholics in the United States alone), along with its other physically and psychologically damaging effects, can lead to excessive facial flushing from the dilation of the small blood vessels in the skin. After many years of repeated flushing episodes in predisposed individuals, the tiny blood vessels can lose their ability to constrict, forming a dense network of disfiguring reddish-purplish marks over the cheeks and nose, known as telangiectasia (see chapter 9).

All drugs with abuse potential, including so-called recreational drugs, have been associated with ill effects on the skin. Tranquilizers and "downers" can cause allergic reactions resulting in skin shedding. Barbiturates can cause blisters around the mouth and on the hips and ankles. "Uppers" (crack, cocaine, speed, and amphetamines) can cause severely dry, chapped lips and allergic rashes. Marijuana can cause hives and reddened eyes and may aggravate acne; it has even been associated with instances of hair loss. Amyl nitrites ("rush," "poppers," "sniffers"), by interfering with proper oxygenation of the skin, can temporarily give it a bluish coloration. Sniffing glue can irritate and peel the skin around the nose and cause oozing; sniffing cocaine can lead to perforation of the cartilage in the nose, leaving a hole between the nostrils. Heroin abuse, which has recently seen a resurgence, has been associated with loss of skin elasticity, making one appear older, and more wrinkled, with dark circles under the eyes. If you have an alcohol or drug problem, seek help before it is too late.

3

In Search of Silky Smooth Skin: Moisturizers

Moisturizers, also called emollients and lubricants, are big business, inviting some of the most inflated claims and wildest advertising hype. Sometimes the ads play on sexual innuendo; other times they purport to be clinical and factual. Moisturizers are frequently described in such alluring terms as "deep energizing," "nourishing," "toning," "pore-shrinking," "skin-firming," "antiaging," "antiwrinkling," "cellular-activating," and "cellular-energizing," to name just a few. In response to (or in spite of) these ad campaigns, consumers spend in excess of $2 billion annually for moisturizers alone ($1.7 billion of which is for facial creams), which range in price from less than $1 per ounce to $125 per ounce or more.

A moisturizer may be defined as any cosmetic that serves to soothe, smooth, and soften your skin and reduce frictional irritation—nothing more. The key word in the definition is *cosmetic*. According to FDA regulations, a cosmetic is defined as any product whose purpose is solely to enhance or beautify the skin. This contrasts sharply with the definition of a topical medication, which is a product that affects the structure and function of your skin. The difference between the two is crucial and has important medical and legal ramifications that are discussed more fully in chapter 6. For our purposes, what it means is that if you are expecting anything more from a conventional moisturizer than softer, smoother skin, you will surely be disappointed. No matter what you have heard or read, and no matter how much you pay for them, moisturizers do not add moisture to your skin nor can they retard or reverse the skin-aging process. All the same, for most people the regular use of moisturizers for the prevention of dryness and irritation and for the maintenance of smooth, supple skin constitutes an extremely important part of a proper skin care regime.

DO YOU NEED A MOISTURIZER?

Some of the most frequently asked questions I hear from my patients relate to moisturizers: Do I need them? Which ones are best? How often should I use them? And so forth.

The fact is, not everyone needs to use a moisturizer. Naturally, people with oily skin are less likely to need them under ordinary circumstances. The decision as to what type of moisturizer you use (if any), as well as how much and how often, depends upon your particular skin type and your lifestyle.

As a rule, I routinely recommend emollients for older people, whose skin generally tends to be drier. But persons of any age who are exposed to prolonged periods of cold, chapping outdoor weather, to indoor heating that drops the relative humidity to below 40 percent in the winter, or to air-conditioned rooms and chlorine pools in the summer, may also benefit from them. Dryness can also be a problem for people who live year-round in arid desert climates. Frequent sun exposure, overzealous skin cleansing, or the use of harsh or alkaline soaps, scrub brushes, or irritating cosmetics may likewise necessitate the use of moisturizers.

Additionally, there are a number of medical conditions and treatments that can dry or irritate the skin and for which moisturizers, along with other therapies, are often recommended. Acne medications, whether for teenage acne or for adult acne, even when used properly, often leave the skin on the dry side. Moisturizers can help and are frequently recommended by dermatologists as part of the overall treatment regimen. Diuretics ("water pills"), commonly used for treating high blood pressure and other forms of heart disease, premenstrual fluid accumulation, and inappropriately for "crash" dieting, may deplete the skin of moisture, Here, too, moisturizers can help. Similarly, people with a predisposition to eczema or psoriasis, two skin conditions affecting millions of people worldwide, also suffer with dry skin problems that require the regular use of moisturizers.

SKIN TYPES

In chapter 2, we examined skin types as they relate to sun sensitivity and the need for sun protection. In the following section, a different skin-typing system is explained, which is important for choosing and using moisturizers and skin cleansers. You are probably already somewhat familiar with this classification, as it is often used at sales counters, facial salons, and in cosmetics advertisements. Skin types include normal skin, dry skin, oily skin, combination skin, and sensitive skin. In determining your skin type, keep in mind that the characteristics of your skin can vary with such factors as your age, the season of the year, climatic changes, air quality, pregnancy, medical illness, or emotional stress.

Normal Skin

As the designation suggests, normal skin means a smooth, supple surface, few if any breakouts, an otherwise clear complexion, and a satisfactory oil/moisture balance.

In general, normal skin results from a complex interaction among three major skin elements: its natural water content, protective oil layer, and the amounts of substances called natural moisturizing factors that are present. Of these, your skin's water content is by far the most important determinant of skin texture; it is the skin's topmost horny layer, normally containing somewhere between 10 and 30 percent water, which is most crucial for maintaining optimal moisture balance. The second factor, your skin's natural protective oil layer or lipid film, which locks in your skin's moisture and prevents its evaporation, is derived from secretions of the oil (sebaceous) glands and from substances derived from the dead cells of the horny layer. The third component, its natural moisturizing factors (NMF), are substances produced by the body that are capable of drawing water upward from the dermis to the skin surface, where it is most needed.

Dry Skin

Dry skin is by far the most common skin affliction. It has been estimated that in the course of our lifetimes, every single one of us will be affected by it to varying degrees. Aging skin is particularly prone to dryness. Mild dryness is characterized by the presence of a fine flakiness to the skin. More severely affected skin appears rough and typically has coarser and more adherent scales and flakes, and by a dull matte finish when makeup is applied. With severe dryness, you can generate showers of flakes by simply rubbing or scratching your skin. Dermatologists often use the terms *xerosis* or *asteatosis* to refer to any severe dry skin condition.

Much remains to be learned about why some people have drier skin than others. Common to all forms of dry skin seems to be an abnormal shedding of cells from the horny layer of the skin. Under ordinary circumstances, single cells are continually being shed from this layer, but in "dry" skin conditions, tightly bound clumps of cells are shed instead. The formation of itchy and painful skin splits and cracks (fissures), profound irritation, eczema, unusual sensitivity to cold, and even infections are among the potential complications of prolonged dry skin problems.

Surprisingly, dry skin is not due to a lack of oils, and there is little evidence that "dry" skin contains substantially less water than normal skin, although there is a slow, progressive decline in skin water content as we age. Nevertheless, individuals with rough, spikey, scaly-looking skin do find their condition worsened by anything that encourages additional fluid loss from the skin surface and improved by adding water and moisturizers.

Although some advertisers try to make you believe otherwise, dryness is not responsible for the development of wrinkles or premature skin aging. So don't expect your wrinkles to disappear permanently by simply using a moisturizer. Dryness can, however, accentuate fine wrinkles if you have already developed them from sun damage or other factors.

Oily Skin

As the designation suggests, this skin type is characterized by a greasy appearance and feel. Individuals with this skin type typically demonstrate an extra shine to their skin, particularly on the forehead and chin, and complain that no matter how much they wash during the day, their skin turns greasy again in no time. The oiliness is often accompanied by enlarged, visible pores, blackheads, and acne. Although the skin may also appear somewhat pallid, premature wrinkling is seldom a problem.

Combination Skin

Given the complexities of the human body, it should hardly come as a surprise that different areas of your face can have different skin types. Combination skin refers to the common situation in which your skin can be oily on the forehead, nose, and chin, the so-called T-zone (because of its shape), but dry around the cheeks, eyes, and mouth. The terms *combination skin* and *T-zone* are favorite buzzwords of facialists and makeup manufacturers.

Sensitive Skin

Sensitive skin is defined as skin that is easily irritated. Since women use cosmetics, they are more likely to recognize the problem than men are, and about 40 percent of women worldwide do complain of this problem. Typically, they complain of burning, stinging, or itching when just about anything is applied to their skin, including soaps, cleansers, moisturizers, and cosmetics. Their skin also tends to react unfavorably to a variety of other factors, including perspiration, changes in temperature, the use of saunas and steam rooms, and the consumption of hot drinks and alcohol. Occasionally, sensitive skin can appear red and inflamed; more often, it appears normal, despite the burning and stinging sensations. Although it tends to be more common among fair-skinned people who blush easily, sensitive skin can be found in people with any skin type. A family trait predisposition is the most likely underlying cause of this problem.

WHAT'S IN MOISTURIZERS?

Nowadays, conventional moisturizers are composed primarily of one or both of two types of ingredients: occlusive ingredients and humectants. Occlusive ingredients are those that, when applied to the skin, lock in the moisture already there and retard its evaporation. Humectants are substances that attract water up from the lower levels of the skin to the horny layer, where it is most needed. These ingredients are most commonly formulated into creams or lotion bases. (A lotion is simply a cream to which more water has been added to make the final product lighter and to enable it go on more smoothly and easily.)

OCCLUSIVE INGREDIENTS

Occlusive ingredients include animal fats, vegetable oils, mineral oils, and silicone oil derivatives. Animal fats include lanolin, mink, turtle, and codfish oils. Lanolin, which is a derivative of sheep oil glands, and anhydrous wool fat, a lanolin derivative, are common ingredients in many moisturizers. Unfortunately, lanolin or its derivatives may clog pores and trigger acne breakouts, and people with sensitive skin are frequently allergic to these substances. The case is very much the same for mink and turtle oils, although manufacturers have tried to play upon the subtle association between the richness of mink coats or the longevity of turtles to market such products.

Olive, safflower, corn, wheat germ, palm kernel, apricot, and sesame seed oils are all examples of common vegetable oils found in many moisturizers. In general, these polyunsaturated oils make satisfactory occlusive ingredients. However, they are generally not as effective as animal fats or mineral oils. In the case of vegetable oils, product manufacturers attempt to link subliminally the known health benefits of consuming polyunsaturated oils for your heart to their benefits for your skin. When it comes to skin, however, vegetable oils offer no special benefits.

Cocoa butter is another commonly employed vegetable-based moisturizer. A solid fat derivative of the roasted seeds of the cacao tree (the source of chocolate and cocoa), cocoa butter melts at room temperature. Although it is an effective moisturizing ingredient, I seldom recommend it because it can irritate sensitive skin.

Plain mineral oil and petroleum derivatives are examples of mineral oils. Used for more than a hundred years, plain petroleum jelly, or petrolatum, is an excellent occlusive moisturizer. Even today, it remains the paradigm of occlusive moisturizers against whose effectiveness all other newly developed moisturizers are compared. It is also very inexpensive and rarely causes allergies. If you have extremely sensitive skin and are easily irritated by most commercial moisturizers, you might try plain petroleum jelly (Vaseline).

Despite its efficacy, petrolatum remains unpopular for some good reasons. Most people find it much too greasy and messy to use regularly, especially during the day; it can also clog pores and trigger acne flare-ups. Fortunately, these days cosmetic chemists have been able to formulate elegant, nongreasy petrolatum-containing moisturizers (such as Curel lotion) that have eliminated many of the drawbacks of the unenhanced product.

Finally, simethicone and dimethicone, two silicone derivatives, have proven themselves excellent occlusive ingredients and are enjoying increasing popularity. Because they are not technically oils, these ingredients are found in many moisturizers that are labeled oil-free, nongreasy, and noncomedogenic. True allergy to these ingredients is quite uncommon, making them a good choice for sensitive skin.

It is important to keep in mind that moisturizers differ not only in the kinds of oils they contain, but in the proportions of oil and water in them. Water-based (oil-in-water) moisturizers contain more water than oil, whereas oil-based moisturizers (water-in-oil) contain more oil than water. Ninety percent of all moisturizers on the market today are of the water-based type. As mentioned earlier, oil-free moisturizers may contain synthetic moisturizers in place of oil. For a quick way to get a sense of whether a moisturizer is water- or oil-based, rub a small amount on the back of your hand. Those that are water-based will cool your skin as the water in them evaporates; those that are oil-based will warm your skin by absorbing the heat.

HUMECTANTS

Glycerin, propylene glycol, butylene glycol, urea, lactic acid, lecithin, and sodium pyrollidone carboxylic acid (PCA) are all examples of common humectants. Humectants are now used widely in many moisturizers, either alone or in combination with occlusive ingredients and alpha hydroxy acids (see chapter 6). They are particularly helpful for loosening scales and dealing with stubborn dry skin problems. They do not provoke acne and, in fact, are particularly useful for countering the drying effects of many topical anti-acne medications.

ADDITIVES OF DOUBTFUL VALUE

Certain ingredients that are included in moisturizers add much to the hype and a lot to the price but little to the benefit of the product. These include collagen, pro-collagen, elastin, hyaluronic acid, amino acids, proteins, DNA, aloe vera, allantoin, algae, vegetable extracts, placental extracts, amniotic fluid extracts, hormones, liposomes, eggs, milk, honey, and royal bee jelly.

Although amino acids, collagen, elastin, hyaluronic acid, and DNA are the building blocks of the body, these substances, when applied to the skin, cannot get in; they cannot be "eaten" or "drunk up" by the skin, as manufacturers would like you to believe. Their molecules are simply too large to penetrate the skin. So despite the inflated claims, any moisturizer products containing these substances are actually no more effective than the occlusive ingredients or humectants that are also contained in them. While you may find that moisturizers containing collagen, elastin, or hyaluronic acid spread more smoothly and have a satiny feel, they don't moisturize any better. These substances may also add some humectant properties, but, in my opinion, products containing them are not worth their often considerably higher prices.

Collagen in moisturizers must not be confused with the injectable collagen preparations Zyderm and Zyplast used by dermatologists for treating wrinkles and depressed scars (see chapter 11). With Zyderm and Zyplast, the collagen material is injected into the deeper level of the skin with a needle precisely where it is needed.

Moisturizers containing hormones usually incorporate very small amounts of estrogens, which may act like humectants in attracting water. The amounts are usually so small that the moisturizer remains categorized as a cosmetic rather than as a drug. But it is precisely because they contain so little hormones that these moisturizers have proven of little benefit. Likewise, placental and amniotic fluid extracts, which supposedly supplement the skin's vitamin and hormone content, are of doubtful value. Here, manufacturers take advantage of the mistaken notion that, since the amnion and placenta nourish the developing embryo, extracts of them can nourish and rejuvenate aging skin.

Herbal additives, such as algae, aloe vera, allantoin, and a variety of herbal extracts, have also gotten their play. Algae (a simple form of plant life), aloe vera (an extract from the succulent aloe plant leaf), and extracts of almond, avocado, cucumber, camomile, jojoba, ginseng, lime, lemon, peach, and wheat-germ, among others, may also be found in moisturizers. Although the use of herbals and vegetable extracts may sound natural and appealing, none of these additives has been demonstrated to impart any significant benefits to moisturizers. The same applies to allantoin, a colorless crystal derived from uric acid, which is touted for its ability to soften skin.

Liposomes, specially synthesized microscopic capsules made from fatty substances, are one of the newest entrants into marketplace. At the present time, research continues into their use for delivering medications to various organs and tissues. Some success has been achieved when they are used for injectable medications. However, in skin preparations, their benefits remain unproven. For the time being, liposome-containing moisturizers represent little more than another expensive allure.

A potpourri of other ingredients—including such items as eggs, milk, honey, and royal bee jelly—have also had their advocates through the years. These ingredients may give a moisturizer a smoother consistency or a lusher look, but that's all. They may be natural and nourishing when eaten, but they do little for you when applied to your skin.

CHOOSING THE RIGHT MOISTURIZER

At last count, the marketplace and cosmetic counters were flooded with more than three hundred fifty brands of general moisturizers and several hundred other special moisturizers for the face. Given the enormous number of claims and testimonials for the success of one cream or another and the wide disparity in retail prices between products, the simple act of purchasing a moisturizer can make your head spin. To confound the matter further, manufacturers produce specific moisturizers for almost every area of your body. There are moisturizers intended only for your face, moisturizers for only around the eyes, and moisturizers for the rest of your body. There are also heavier night creams and lighter day creams.

Fortunately, to find a product that's right for you, you need only know your skin type and follow a few simple guidelines. The moisturizer you choose should be convenient to purchase and should be available at your local supermarket or corner drugstore, not just sold at the so-called finest department stores. It should cost no more than a few dollars for several fluid ounces, so that you can use it liberally, if necessary. You don't generally need separate moisturizers for each area of your skin or, for that matter, one moisturizer for day and another for night. Although about 75 percent of moisturizers contain fragrances, you should avoid fragranced products, since they add nothing to the lubricating benefits of a moisturizer and add considerably to its potential for causing irritation or allergy. If you desire a particular scent, the use of a separate perfume or cologne applied only to the few spots where you want it is a better approach, since perfumes in moisturizers, by virtue of their being applied to larger areas of your skin, are more likely to cause problems.

For best effect, apply moisturizers to damp skin, immediately after washing, to replace the natural oils stripped by washing and drying and to lock in the moisture absorbed while washing. You should also use them regularly rather than sporadically, as part of a daily skin care routine.

If you have normal skin, you may not need a moisturizer at all, but if you do, a light, hypoallergenic, preservative-free, all-purpose water-based moisturizer, such as Carmol-10 lotion will probably do just fine for daily use.

If you have dry or flaky skin, you may also find the kind of moisturizer just mentioned to be satisfactory for your needs. However, if your skin is exceptionally dry, you might try a slightly heavier oil-based cream formulation or even plain petroleum jelly for night use, if you can tolerate the greasiness and messiness. Alternatively, you might try Carmol-20 cream, which contains 20 percent urea, a potent humectant. This agent is effective in dealing with stubborn dry skin and works to soften the skin and to dissolve rough, dry patches.

If you have oily, acne-prone skin, you may not need moisturizers, but if occasionally you do, or if anti-acne medications are overly drying your skin, choose water-based or oil-free products, preferably in lotion form. Look for products that are specifically labeled *nonacnegenic* (products that do not provoke acne) or *noncomedogenic* (products that do not stimulate blackheads or whiteheads), to indicate that at least some testing has been done to determine that they do not do so. In addition, you should avoid moisturizers containing the following potential acne-aggravating ingredients: isopropyl myristate, isopropyl esters, oleic acid, stearic acid, lanolin and lanolin derivatives, heavy mineral oil, linseed oil, olive oil, and cocoa butter.

If you have combination skin, don't rely on products that claim that they can handle dryness and oiliness at the same time. A one-product-does-both usually doesn't do either job very well. Besides, it is very difficult to understand how any product can "know" to use its drying ingredients only on your oily areas and its oilier ingredients in your dry areas. Instead, you should deal with your drier patches as described above, after which you may more easily treat your entire face with products intended for oily skin.

If you have sensitive skin, selecting any product can be difficult. A good rule of thumb is the fewer the ingredients, the better. This means trying a light, hypoallergenic (see chapter 5), fragrance-free moisturizer, such as fragrance-free Curel lotion, and testing it on a small area for a few days. You might, for example, start by applying it only to a small area behind your ears for a few days to be sure that you do not experience an adverse reaction. You may have to test several products in this fashion, but once you have found a product that works for you and does not irritate, sting, or burn, stick with it.

4

Coming Clean: Selecting the Right Cleansers

After adequate sun protection and appropriate moisturization, proper cleansing is the third important aspect of keeping your skin healthier and younger-looking. Every day, your skin interacts with dirt, pollution, cosmetics, oils, dead skin cells, and perspiration, and the main reason for washing is to get rid of these things. But for most people, rinsing with plain water is not sufficient, because heavy, greasy substances, like cosmetics and dirt, repel water and are difficult to remove without some help. That's where soaps and other cleansers come in. All soaps and cleansers work by dissolving grease so that it can be rinsed off with water. The ideal cleanser must walk a fine line between being able to take off just the unwanted greases while leaving your natural oils and natural moisturizing factors intact. To date, no cleanser is able to do this perfectly.

Despite the claims of some soap manufacturers, cleansers cannot rejuvenate your skin or make you younger-looking in any number of days, nor can they fight wrinkles or give your complexion that "special glow" or blush. To the contrary, rather than being "soothing" or "gentle on your skin," soaps and cleansers are, by their very nature, to some degree irritating. Cleaning your skin and leaving it freshened are the sole functions of all cleansers.

HOW THEY WORK

To clean, soaps and detergents employ chemicals called emulsifiers or surfactants, substances whose molecules have the ability to attract and simultaneously hold on to both oil and water, thereby making it possible for greasy environmental substances and skin oils to be soaped up and rinsed away with plain water. Without these agents, it would be like trying to clean petroleum jelly from your hands by simply running them under the tap; the water would just form beads on the surface and run off.

YOUR OPTIONS

Consumers these days are confronted with many choices of facial cleansers: old-fashioned toilet soaps, superfatted soaps, soapless soaps (synthetic detergent soaps or "syndets"), cleansing creams and lotions, washable creams and lotions, soaps with special additives, and astringents. While the overall cleansing performance and effectiveness of each of these items varies little, the retail prices of the various brands of cleansers may differ dramatically. Bar soaps, for example, may range from less than twenty cents per bar to nearly nine dollars per bar, where packaging and fragrance account for about 30 percent of the retail price. They may also differ in durability, that is, how slowly or quickly a particular brand of soap melts away in your soap dish. And while they may also differ in how richly they lather, it is not actually necessary for a cleanser to lather well in order to be effective.

In the final analysis, your choice of cleanser should take into account your particular skin type and your individual needs. It will most likely also be influenced by advertising allure and your personal preferences for product color, fragrance, feel, and flair for luxury.

TOILET SOAPS

Toilet soap, which is available in opaque bars, is basically plain old-fashioned soap composed of the salts of animal or vegetable fats and olive oils (tallow). Palm kernel or coconut oils are often added to enhance lathering. About half of all currently available toilet soaps are milled soaps, meaning that the ingredients and additives have been thoroughly and evenly blended and the bars compressed by machinery to remove all excess moisture.

In general, toilet soaps are inexpensive and clean satisfactorily. On the other hand, they tend to be rather alkaline and thus have the potential to be irritating. Overuse can be especially irritating, in that it affects the skin's normal acid mantle. Toilet soaps have the additional disadvantage that when they are combined with hard water (water containing naturally high amounts of calcium or magnesium minerals), sticky, scummy, irritating residues form in the sink basin and on your skin. In hard water areas, the use of water softeners or synthetic detergent soaps are good alternatives. Ivory Soap is probably the best-known brand of plain soap.

SUPERFATTED SOAPS

Superfatted soaps are essentially toilet soaps to which moisturizers such as cold cream, lanolin, mineral oil, olive oil, cocoa butter, or other neutral fats have been added. The amount of fatty material added varies widely among different brands. While most soaps ordinarily contain less than 2 percent fat, superfatted soaps usually contain between 5 and 15 percent fat. The fatty moisturizers in superfatted soaps are intended to counter the degreasing effects of the soap—a difficult task to actually accomplish. Many people do prefer these soaps, finding them more gentle on their skin. On the other hand, others complain that they deposit a greasy residue on the skin and that the soaps melt too quickly in the soap dish. (Oilatum is an example of a superfatted soap.) Transparent soaps are special forms of superfatted soaps, which—in addition to a higher fat content, often in the form of castor oil or resin—contain glycerin (at least 10 percent more than in other soaps), alcohol, and sugar. The glycerin is responsible for the soft consistency and transparency of these products. (Neutrogena soap is a well-known brand in this category.)

SOAPLESS SOAPS

Also called synthetic detergent soaps ("syndets"), or soap-free cleansers, these products are derived from petroleum materials, fatty acids, and other substances. Cosmetic and pharmaceutical chemists have formulated these to be satisfactory cleansers and to be less alkaline and less irritating than plain soaps. They also do not leave residues on your skin or in the sink in hard water areas and don't leave a greasy aftereffect to the skin as do the super-fatted soaps. Unlike transparent soaps, they tend to lather reasonably well and usually do not melt so easily in the soap dish. For these reasons, I prefer these cleansers and generally recommend products such as fragrance- and dye-free Formula 405 Facial and Body Cleanser for the majority of my patients.

WASHABLE LOTIONS AND LIQUID SOAPS

Washable creams and lotions have many of the same ingredients as bar soaps. However, they generally tend to be more expensive than bar soaps. Heavy on their moisturizing content, these products may be thought of as moisturizers to which soaps or detergents have been added. Like other cleansers, they are intended to be rinsed off with water. Washable lotions are simply creams to which more water has been added to make them thinner and more easily spreadable.

Some of the major cosmetic manufacturers seem to be focusing their attention on liquid soaps, which are heavier on their soap or detergent content than are washable lotions. In addition, they usually contain glycerin. Liquid soaps are formulated to be rinsed off with water. They possess no particular advantage over their bar counterparts, although they come in convenient pump dispensers. Oil of Olay's Sensitive Skin Foaming Facial Wash is a good example.

Washable lotions and liquid soaps should not be confused with cleansing creams or lotions, which are essentially moisturizers used for cleaning purposes. They are meant to be applied and then wiped off with a facial tissue or soft towel, rather than washed off with water. Liquefying creams are simply cleansing creams that contain oils and waxes that melt upon contact with skin heat. Otherwise, they differ little from cleansing creams and have no special properties.

Like many other moisturizers, cleansing lotions and liquefying creams tend to be greasy and can leave a film on your skin. And because they contain little or no detergent, they generally clean poorly. They are most useful for removing makeup, particularly oil-based or heavy theater makeups and powders. Because you generally need to follow their use with a gentle soap and water cleansing to feel clean, most of their supposed value is mitigated.

DEODORANT SOAPS

Under ordinary circumstances, deodorant soaps have little place in facial skin care. Their primary function is to suppress odor-producing bacteria and to mask body odor. To do so, they contain two major types of ingredients: antiseptics (either triclosan or triclocarban) for suppressing bacteria, and perfumes for masking odor. Since neither bacteria nor odor is really a problem in facial skin, the additives in deodorant soaps merely increase the potential for irritation and allergy, and for that reason they should ordinarily be avoided unless otherwise recommended by your dermatologist.

FANCY ADDITIVES

Over the years, a variety of ingredients have been added to soaps in an attempt to improve them or increase their allure. These include an array of so-called organic, herbal, or other natural additives, medications and abrasives. The truth is that fruit, vegetable, and herbal soaps clean no better than conventional soaps and provide no additional benefits. Moreover, during the soap-manufacturing process, the herbs, fruits, or vegetable additives become so strained, sterilized, alcohol-purified, and mixed with preservatives that by the time the entire process is complete, the end product needs to have artificial colorings and fragrances just to simulate the real thing. And the more chemicals there are, the greater the possibility for causing irritation or allergy.

Medicated soaps are cleansers that contain topical drugs in addition to the cleansing agent. Depending upon the particular conditions for which they are recommended, these products may contain sulfur, resorcinol, salicylic acid, benzoyl peroxide, or antiseptics. The concept may seem good, but to be of value, a medication must remain in contact with your skin for an extended period of time, something that soaps, which are rinsed off quickly, do not do. In general, medicated soaps tend to be more drying and more irritating than conventional cleansers. If you have a specific skin condition, see your dermatologist.

Abrasive cleansers, or exfoliating cleansers, contain tiny particles or grains that are supposed to abrade your skin mildly, slough off the surface layer of dead cells, and leave your skin with a smooth, glowing complexion. Some abrasive soaps may contain as much as 25 percent pumice (ground volcanic rock). For many people, they can be excessively harsh and drying and should be used with great care. Overzealous use, especially if combined with certain potent anti-acne medications, can leave your skin extremely dry, flaky, or even cracked; in extreme cases, "broken" blood vessels may even result. Here, too, I suggest that you consult your physician before resorting to these products.

Astringents, fresheners, clarifying lotions, and toners are products intended to freshen and cleanse the skin and "shrink" pores. In fact, these items do little more than blot oiliness and make your face feel cool, tight, and tingly. Any pore "shrinkage" resulting from their use is due to irritation of the opening of the pores and is only temporary, generally lasting no more than three hours after use. All three products are basically composed of water, alcohol, and fragrances, to which menthol, witch hazel, or camphor may be added to impart the tingly sensation, and mint, eucalyptus, and lemon added for fragrance. None of these additives, however, confers any special properties. Some people with excessively oily skin, especially during hot, humid weather, may find astringents helpful for blotting up oiliness. Persons with combination skin may also find astringents useful for the T-zone between washings. For most people, however, a thorough soap-and-water cleansing is probably sufficient. If you wish to use astringents, do so as infrequently as possible to prevent overdryness and irritation. If you have naturally dry, sensitive skin or are being treated with drying, anti-acne medications, you may find astringents too irritating and should probably avoid them altogether, particularly during the winter months.

Selecting What's Right for You

For individuals with normal skin, most soaps or cleansers will probably do. Even after they use harsher alkaline soaps, the natural skin acidity of these lucky individuals generally returns to normal very shortly after rinsing.

If you have oily skin, you may find the regular use of toilet soaps satisfactory. For extremely oily skin, especially during hot and humid weather, consider supplementing your morning and night cleansing with a midmorning or midafternoon application of an astringent to blot up the excess oiliness. Astringent pads, such as Stridex, are convenient to carry with you. You may alternatively find abrasive soaps to be useful, but these should only be used occasionally, to minimize potential irritation. However, you should be especially cautious with abrasive cleansers if you have acne or other types of inflammation, since they may aggravate your condition.

If you have combination skin, you may want to clean your face with a gentle cleanser and then later in the day additionally cleanse the T-zone with an astringent, preferably one that is alcohol-free, as needed. Or if you like, you may want to use a soap-free cleanser on the dryer, outer areas of your face and a toilet soap on the oilier T-zone region, although many people find this a bit inconvenient.

When it comes to cleansers, dry and sensitive skin types have very similar needs. If you have either type, or if you are using drying acne medications, you will probably find a basic toilet soap too irritating for routine use. A soap-free, sensitive-skin cleanser would be your best bet. Be cautious with transparent soaps: Because of their higher glycerin and alcohol content, they may draw water from the skin and may thus be too drying. They may be more useful for the occasional individual with sensitive but oily skin.

For more troublesome dry or sensitive skin, washable lotions can sometimes be helpful. For example, you might try alternating the use of a sensitive-skin bar and a washable lotion, cleansing with the bar in the morning and using the washable lotion at night. Or you might use the bar one day and a washable lotion the next, depending upon your needs. Finally, if you have extremely dry or sensitive skin and absolutely cannot tolerate any form of soap or detergent cleanser, you should consider the use of cleansing creams and lotions.

CLEANSING TIPS

The use of strong soaps, hot water, and super-scrubbing were at one time the cleansing prescriptions of the day. However, scientific thinking on this matter has changed during the last decade or so. Vigorous scrubbing with soap and hot water are no longer routinely advised and are best reserved for getting greasy dinner plates squeaky-clean. Gentle cleansing is the new order. To prevent stripping your skin of its oils and natural moisturizing factors, avoid using polyester scrub sponges or washclothes (use just your fingertips), and keep the water tepid rather than very hot. After lathering, rinse thoroughly with plenty of water to remove any potentially irritating soapy debris, lightly pat your skin dry (do not rub), and then apply your moisturizer (while your skin is still damp, rather than completely dry). If you want your cleansing dollars to go further, remove bars from the soap dish and dry them after each use or purchase a soap dish with a built-in drain.

5

Making the Most
of Makeup

The average woman uses fifteen different cosmetics every single day, making these products big business. Roughly $3 billion is spent annually on skin-care cosmetics, mostly by women, and this figure is expected to continue climbing at a rate of about 7 percent a year. What guides someone to select one brand over another is often a matter of individual preference for fragrance, color, feel, packaging, or simply the result of successful marketing. However, since different brands intended for the same purposes and having many of the same active ingredients often differ sharply in price, making the best choices for your money can be an important issue. To select wisely, you need to know your skin type (see chapter 3) and some basics about cosmetic ingredients and marketing claims.

COSMETIC INGREDIENTS

Cosmetic chemistry is a highly complex field, and a glance at almost any cosmetic ingredient label is usually enough to make the uninitiated feel overwhelmed and confused. At the very least, you should be aware that by law, product ingredients are listed on cosmetic product labels in the order of their relative amounts within the makeup. This means that even without knowing how much of a particular ingredient a product contains, you do at least know that it contains more of those ingredients listed first on the label than those listed last.

Another major step to being a better consumer is knowing which ingredients in a cosmetic were put there to benefit you and which are there to either preserve the product or benefit the manufacturer. Those ingredients put there to help you are the active ingredients; those needed for the manufacture of the product or to prevent spoiling may be thought of as the inactive ingredients. Any ingredients put there to increase sales appeal or advertising hype (and that are of no proven medical value) may be considered unnecessary additives. A quick glance at Table 2 can help you to separate the active from the inactive and unnecessary ingredients when purchasing cosmetics.

To make the table more comprehensible, you need to familiarize yourself with a few definitions. Emollients, as you may recall from chapter 3, are chemicals used to soften and smooth your skin. Humectants are substances that absorb moisture from the air and also lock moisture in the skin. Solvents, the best example of which is plain water, are carrier liquids into which other ingredients are dissolved. Emulsifying agents help oil and water to stay mixed in lotions and creams. Emulsion stabilizers keep oil and water from separating. Preservatives, antioxidants, and chemical stabilizers prolong shelf life by suppressing germs and preventing unwanted chemical reactions. Thickening, stiffening, and suspending agents and viscosity builders are used to give a "cushiony" feel to products and to thicken their consistency. Gellants are thickeners that form transparent gels when combined with alchohol, acetone, or water. Powder formers are used to formulate powdery products.

In the complex world of cosmetic chemistry, many ingredients serve more than one purpose. It should be obvious that an expensive cosmetic bearing a label of a long list of ingredients with tongue-twisting chemical names may not necessarily be better than its less-expensive competitors that have the same active ingredients.

When you are deciding among several products used for the same purpose, you need only compare their active ingredients, and unless you know that you are allergic to one or the other, you may basically ignore the inactive and unnecessary ones. For example, when looking to buy a moisturizer, be aware that the active ingredients are its moisturizing and humectant ingredients, which serve to soften and smooth your skin. In the case of foundation makeup, the active ingredients are the pigments (colors), which give you the color and shade, and the moisturizers, which allow the colors to be applied more smoothly and evenly. Evaluating cosmetics in this way can be less bewildering than attempting to make sense of product labels often containing twenty or more ingredients.

Try it for yourself the next time you are at the cosmetics counter. Compare two or three products with the same function but that differ a great deal in price. (For example, you might compare under-makeup moisturizers or foundation makeups.) You will probably find that all three products contain the same active ingredients (all will have the same ingredients listed first on the label. Toward the end of the ingredient list, you will also probably find one or more unnecessary ingredients, such as collagen, aloe vera, or algae, which are being touted for their supposed abilities to keep your skin younger or healthier. Along with fancier packaging, the addition of unnecessary ingredients is largely responsible for the higher prices. I'm not saying that it's not okay to buy more expensive cosmetics when you like the look or feel of

Table 2

Common Cosmetic Ingredients, by Function

ACTIVE INGREDIENTS

EMOLLIENTS

Butyl stearate
Caprylic/capric triglyceride
Castor oil
Cetearyl alcohol
Cetyl alcohol
Diisopropyl adipate
Glycerin
Glyceryl monostearate
Isopropyl myristate
Isopropyl palmitate
Lanolin
Lanolin alcohol
Lanolin, hydrogenated
Mineral oil
Petrolatum
Polyethylene glycols
Polyoxethylene lauryl ether
Polyoxypropylene 15 stearyl ether
Propylene glycol stearate
Silicone
Squalane
Stearic acid

Steryl alcohol
Vegetable oils

HUMECTANTS

Glycerin
Lactic acid
Lecithin
Propylene glycol
Sorbitol solution
Urea

COMMON PIGMENTS (COLORS)

Bismuth oxychloride
Carmine
Chromium oxide green
D&C and FD&C Colors
Ferric ammonium ferrocyanide
Ferric ferrocyanide
Iron oxides
Manganese violet
Mica
Titanium dioxide (white pigment)
Ultramarine blue

INACTIVE INGREDIENTS

EMULSIFYING AGENTS
(SURFACTANTS)

Amphoteric-9
Carbomer
Cetearyl alcohol (and)
  ceteareth-20
Cholesterol
Disodium monooleamido-
  sulfosuccinate

Emulsifying wax, NF
Lanolin
Lanolin alcohol (laureths)
Lanolin, hydrogenated
Lecithin
Polyethylene glycol 1000
  monocetylether
Polyoxyl 40 stearate
Polysorbates

Sodium laureth sulfate
Sodium lauryl sulfate
Sorbitan esters
Stearic acid
Tea stearate
Trolamine

SOLVENTS

Alcohol
Diisopropyl adipate
Glycerin
1,2,6-hexanetriol
Isopropyl myristate
Polyoxypropylene 15 stearyl ether
Propylene carbonate
Propylene glycol

THICKENING, STIFFENING, AND
SUSPENDING AGENTS

Beeswax
Candelilla, carnauba, and cetyl
   esters wax
Carbomer
Cellulose gums
Dextrin
Mannitol
Ozokerite (ceresin)
Polyethylene
Xanthan gum

PRESERVATIVES, ANTIOXIDANTS,
AND CHEMICAL STABILIZERS

Alcohol and benzyl alcohol
Butylated hydroxyanisole (BHA)
Butylated hydroxytoluene (BHT)
Chlorocresol
Citric and sorbic acid
Edetate disodium (EDTA)
Imidazolidinyl urea
Parabens
Phenylmercuricacetate
Potassium sorbate
Propyl gallate

Propylene glycol
Quarternium-15
Sodium bisulfite
Tocopherol (vitamin E)

EMULSION STABILIZERS AND
VISCOSITY BUILDERS

Carbomer
Cetearyl, cetyl, and stearyl
   alcohol
Glyceryl monostearate
Paraffin
Polyethylene glycols
Propylene glycol stearate

GELLANTS

Carbomer
Carboxymethyl cellulose
Hydroxymethyl cellulose
Methyl cellulose

POWER FORMERS

Bentonite (hydrated aluminum
   silicate clay)
Magnesium aluminum silicate
Magnesium silicate
Magnesium stearate
Talc

ADDITIVES OF UNPROVEN VALUE

Algae
Allantoin
Aloe vera
Collagen
Eggs
Elastin
Flavorings
Fragrances (except in perfumes,
   colognes, and toilet water)
Honey
Hyaluronic acid
Milk
Placental extract
RNA

them. What is important is that you do not do so because you think you're getting more for your money.

COMMON COSMETICS AND THEIR ACTIVE INGREDIENTS

Except for astringents and perfumes, the basic formula for the overwhelming majority of most facial cosmetics are merely variations on the old cold cream (moisturizer) formula, to which pigments or other special active ingredients have been added for particular purposes. Contrary to what many cosmetic manufacturers have you believe, there is no magic to the formulas of these products.

MOISTURIZERS

As you already know, moisturizers (see chapter 3) are cosmetics intended to smooth and soften skin and to lock in its natural water content. Modified—sometimes just a little, sometimes dramatically—to meet a particular need, moisturizers are the vehicles (bases) into which most other makeup ingredients are dissolved or suspended.

All moisturizer formulas are variations of the old formula for cold cream (water, waxes, and oils or fats) and are available as lotions or creams. Oil-free moisturizers contain synthetic oils, usually silicone oils, rather than oils derived from natural substances and so are better for oily or acne-prone skin. Water-based moisturizers, as the designation suggests, contain more water and less oil and are quite good for normal or slightly dry skin types. Oil-based moisturizers, containing more oil than water, are better for dry or sensitive skin. Moisturizers that contain humectants such as lactic acid may be useful for all skin types, although some people with sensitive skin complain of stinging or itching with these products.

MASKS AND PACKS

There are two basic types of masks: cream masks and paste masks. (Occasionally, you will find mask spelled *masque*. A mask and a masque are essentially the same, except that you usually pay more when the product is spelled *masque*.) Both cream and paste masks are supposed to cleanse and refresh your skin, absorb oil, and promote mild peeling.

Cream masks have the basic oil, wax, and water formula of moisturizers. As such, they may aggravate oily or acne-prone skin. Paste masks, on the other hand, are composed of a powdery base to which abrasives such as almond meal, brans, oats, or ground apricot pits have been added for peeling, and bentonite, kaolin (fuller's earth), or magnesium aluminum silicate has been incorporated to thicken these products and enhance their ability to absorb oils. If you have naturally dry or sensitive skin or are being treated with drying acne medications, you are likely to find abrasive paste masks irritating. I rarely recommend the use of either type of mask. Instead, a regular gentle soap-and-water cleansing is more than adequate for removing oils, dirt, and cosmetics. If moisturization is needed, a separate moisturizer may be used after cleansing.

FOUNDATION MAKEUP

Foundations are used to even out skin tones and to act as a base for blushes and eye makeups. In their simplest form, they are moisturizers to which pigments have been added to give them color. Iron oxides and ultramarine blue are examples of common foundation pigments. Depending upon the product, bismuth oxychloride and mica, called pearlizers, may also be added to impart a shimmering, glittering look, and magnesium aluminum silicate or talc incorporated to give a matte finish. Obviously, in these makeups, both the pigments and the moisturizer are considered the active ingredients. If they also contain a sunscreen or sunblocking ingredient, that also must be considered part of the active ingredients.

The selection of the base should be made by your skin type: water-based foundations for normal skin, oil-free foundations for oily or acne-prone skin, and oil-based products for dry skin. If you have combination skin, you are better off applying an under-makeup moisturizer on your dry areas and then applying a foundation intended for oily skin to your entire face. People with sensitive skin should be especially cautious in using foundations containing sunscreens. At those times when you need one, it would be better to use a separate, fragrance-free, moisturizing sunscreen under your makeup. In this way, you can reduce your exposure to sunscreens to only those times when you actually need them.

When choosing a foundation, test for the right color. To do this, apply the foundation to the jawline and attempt to blend it over the edge of your jaw. When looking for the correct shade, many women mistakenly rub the makeup on their palms or wrists. Since the skin color of your palm and wrist usually differs somewhat from your face color, you can get a false impression of the effect this way. If you choose a shade that is closer to the color of your neck, you won't have to apply it there; this means less chance of your foundation rubbing off and staining your clothes.

Sunless Tanning Agents

Artificial tanning agents or sunless tanners have become quite popular lately. Since they require no outdoor exposure in order to work, they are quite safe. Two major types are currently available: bronzers and skin stains. Bronzers are products containing a water-soluble pigment that is deposited on the skin. No chemical reaction occurs between the skin and the colorant, and because they are water-soluble, bronzers can be washed off with soap and water if you don't like the effect. On the other hand, if you are pleased with your tan, it can become a nuisance to have to reapply the product continually. Since bronzers by themselves offer little actual protection from the sun's rays, you must follow the usual sun precautions discussed in chapter 2.

Sunless tanning lotions containing the chemical dihydroxyacetone (DHA) have become extremely popular and are available in creams, lotions, and gels. DHA is a harmless skin dye that chemically binds to your skin and stains the upper part of the horny layer a brown or reddish-brown color. The major advantage of DHA-containing tanning agents as compared to bronzers is that the tan lasts longer, in many cases up to four days. The tan gradually fades as the stained cells of the horny layer are naturally shed or washed away with soap and water.

Being longer-lasting becomes a disadvantage if you happen to dislike the color of your tan. For that reason, I strongly recommend that you apply a tiny test amount to a hidden area of your skin, such as behind the ear. If you like the resulting color, you can then apply it to all desired areas. Most people find that several coats are needed to achieve the desired skin tone. Again, as in the case of bronzers, no matter how deeply tanned you may appear, sunless tanners provide no significant protection from the sun. While a number of products also contain sunscreens, the level of SPF (between 2 and 8) often is not sufficient for most people's needs. It is therefore best to use the sunless tanner at night before retiring and to use a sunscreen in the morning.

MASKING COSMETICS

Masking or camouflaging cosmetics are special foundations available for covering a variety of scars, surface flaws, skin discolorations, postsurgical bruising or skin staining, and other irregularities. Very much like thick, opaque theater makeup, these products are heavier, water-resistant, oil-based foundations containing greater amounts of pigment for better coverage. For covering spot discolorations or irregularities, cover sticks (water-resistant masking foundations in stick form) are available. A higher proportion of waxes is responsible for the thickness and body of these products. They are thick enough to be effective sunblockers and even durable enough to withstand the beach or chlorine swimming. They are also quite useful for individuals with dry skin. But because of the thick oily coverage, either type of masking cosmetic must be used with caution in oily or acne-prone individuals. Three of the more well known brands offering a wide selection of colors include Lydia O'Leary/ Covermark, Dermablend Corrective Cosmetics, and Natural Cover Cosmetics.

CONCEALERS

Concealers, also called primers, neutralizers, or facial undercover cosmetics, are products designed to be worn under facial foundation to blend pigment irregularities. They are generally creamy cosmetics available in three colors: green, yellow, and purple. Green is useful for camouflaging reddish tones, such as ruddy complexions, "broken" blood vessels, or the healing phases after chemical peels (chapter 7) and dermabrasions (chapter 8). Yellow is used to correct bluish skin discolorations, dark circles under the eyes, and pasty complexions. Purple is used to neutralize yellow spots and sallow complexions. Concealers work by restoring discolorations to flesh-color: green + red = brown; yellow + blue = brown; and purple + yellow = brown. While these products are typically lighter than masking cosmetics and are generally suitable for normal to dry skin, they should still be used with caution by oily or acne-prone skin types. Finally, for numerous dark spots or depressed scars, you might try a white, pearlized (mica-containing) micronized titanium dioxide undercover cosmetic, which reflects light and minimizes shadows.

BLUSHES

Blushes or rouges, available in cream or powder varieties, are cosmetics that are used to add color to your face and to provide shading and contour. Cream blushes are composed of pigments suspended in a thick, creamy moisturizing base. For that reason, they tend to clog pores and should be avoided if you are acne-prone. Powder blushes are powder-based cosmetics to which pigments have been added. Because they are oil-absorbent, powder blushes are less likely to aggravate acne, but they may be slightly drying for dry or sensitive skin types.

EYESHADOWS

Eyeshadows are used to provide color, highlights, and shading to the upper eyelids. Like blushes, they come in cream and powder forms. Cream eyeshadows are pigments in an oil/wax moisturizing base, and powder shadows are pigments suspended in a talc-rich, oil/wax–based moisturizer. The absence of water in either type makes these products less likely to run. Titanium dioxide may be added to the basic formula for a matte finish; pearlizers can create a glittery, shimmery look; and powders of metals like copper, aluminum, or silver can create an iridescent look.

EYELINERS

Eyeliners, which are sold in liquid and pencil form, emphasize and define the eyelid margins. Liquid eyeliners are made of wax/oil bases to which pigments and plasticizing chemicals, frequently acrylics or acrylates, have been added to impart luster and give body. Pencil eyeliners contain higher amounts of wax for stiffening the eyeliner into pencil form.

Eyeliners must be handled and applied with care. If applied improperly—too close to the lid margins or too close to the inner eyelids—eyeliner pigments may cause a chemical inflammation of the delicate mucous membranes on the inside of your eyelid. Moreover, if pigment granules embed themselves into the delicate eyelid membranes, they may may permanently tattoo them. Since the concentrations of preservatives in eyeliners are purposely kept low in order to prevent possible eye irritations, you must be especially careful not to contaminate these products with bacteria. To be safe, never share your eye cosmetics with anyone else.

Mascaras

Mascaras are used to add color, definition, and intensity to eyelashes, as well as to lengthen and thicken them. By far the most popular eyelash cosmetic, they are sold in water-based, water-resistant, and waterproof forms. Waterproof mascara, composed of a thick, water-free, oil/wax base to which the desired pigments are added, must be applied with a brush. Water-based products are pigments in a moisturizing, water-in-oil base. Those that are water-resistant contain higher concentrations of wax, acrylates, or shellacs to thicken them and to prevent running. You may remove both the water-based and water-resistant varieties with soap and water, although waterproof mascaras usually require a mineral oil–based cleansing lotion. Mascaras will not cause eyelashes to fall out permanently, as some people needlessly fear. Although loose hairs do come out whenever the product is applied or removed, these hairs grow back.

Lash extender mascaras are liquid mascaras to which synthetic fibers, usually rayon or nylon, are added to coat the natural lashes and "extend" them. If you wear contact lenses, you should avoid lash extender mascaras since corneal scratching or more severe corneal damage can result if the fibers get under the lenses. Talc and kaolin may also be added to mascaras for lash thickening, and if you wear lenses you should exercise similar caution when considering these cosmetics.

LIPSTICKS AND LIP GLOSSES

Lipsticks add color to your lips, and lip glosses add a shine; both products have an oil/wax base. In lipsticks, pigments are added to impart color, and in glosses, sheen-producing ingredients such as lanolin are added. Nowadays, sunscreens, such as PABA or its derivatives, are frequently included in lipsticks to help prevent sun damage to the delicate lips. The fragrances and flavorings that are sometimes added to lip glosses provide no additional benefits and should be considered unnecessary additives.

COLOGNES, TOILET WATER, AND PERFUMES

Colognes contain about 88 to 95 percent alcohol and between 5 and 12 percent fragrance. Perfumes contain about 70 to 80 percent alcohol and 15 to 30 percent fragrance. Toilet waters are intermediate between colognes and perfumes.

Fragrances are extremely complex mixtures of ingredients. There are currently more than ten thousand different chemical essences derived from animal, flower, root, and plant oils, as well as many synthetic fragrances. Fragrances are believed to be responsible for the majority of all adverse reactions to cosmetics. In one large study, cinnamic alcohol, cinnamic aldehyde, hydroxycitronell, musk ambrette, isoeugenol, and geranoil were the essence ingredients most frequently associated with skin reactions.

As a rule, the more alcohol in a product, the shorter its shelf life. Colognes, therefore, are usually good for about six months and the strongest of perfumes for slightly more than a year. To extend their shelf life, your fragrance products should be stored in cool, dark places, since heat and sunlight promote evaporation.

MARKETING CLAIMS

Legally defined, cosmetics are products manufactured for the sole purpose of making you look better. Although topical medications—preparations intended to affect the structure and function of your skin—are subject to stringent FDA regulation, cosmetics escape such regulation. The ramifications of this are of no small importance. For example, although the FDA does insist that the main ingredients be listed on the label of a cosmetic, fragrances or flavorings need not be listed. The FDA likewise does not require efficacy testing for cosmetics. Cosmetics manufacturers need only perform sufficient testing on their products to assure their general safety for use by the public. They are not required to demonstrate that their products actually do for you what the marketing claims say they are supposed to. "In cosmetics," says the FDA, "you are what you claim." Moreover, the terms *hypoallergenic, nonirritating, noncomedogenic, and nonacnegenic*, while used freely to commercialize many different kinds of cosmetics, have no legal or regulatory definition either by the FDA or the FTC, nor is there an industry standard for what these terms mean. The ultimate responsibility for success and satisfaction with any particular cosmetic falls largely into your hands.

Despite the lack of regulations and consensus, however, you may find a working definition of the following terms helpful for guiding you when choosing cosmetics.

HYPOALLERGENIC

Fortunately, true allergic reactions to cosmetics are rare, constituting only about 0.3 percent of all problems seen by dermatologists and only about 5 percent of all types of contact allergies. Such allergies may show up as redness, itching, swelling, and blistering.

Individuals with known contact allergies and those with very sensitive skin often look for products labeled *hypoallergenic*. Despite the fact that many people misinterpret the term to mean "not causing allergies at all," hypoallergenic actually means that a cosmetic manufacturer has taken measures to eliminate from its products ingredients such as perfumes and fragrances that are known to have a greater likelihood of provoking allergies. If you do develop an allergy, you may find that these manufacturers are more likely to help your dermatologist to find the ingredient(s) in their products that may be causing the problem. Many of them will not only provide your doctor with a complete list of ingredients but may also supply sample amounts of these ingredients in a form suitable for allergy testing. I have found the manufacturers of Almay, Allercreme, Clinique, and Revlon hypoallergenic cosmetic lines to be particularly responsible in these areas.

In the United States today, most major cosmetic houses produce hypoallergenic products whether or not they are labeled so—if for no other reason but good business sense. As companies are in business to sell products and make money, no company wants to market a cosmetic that causes allergic reactions so often that few people would consider purchasing it again.

In the event that you do become allergic to a specific brand of cosmetic, you don't necessarily have to give up using all brands of that type of product. With a little experimentation, you may be able to find the specific item that causes you problems, eliminate it, and continue using cosmetics.

Let's say that you developed an allergy to a particular brand of reddish cream blush. The first thing you should do, of course, is stop using the suspected trouble-making blush. Next, wait until the allergy completely clears. This may take one to two weeks. Then choose another brand of reddish cream blush. If after three continuous days of use, you don't develop allergic symptoms to the new blush, it is likely that your allergy is not to the red pigment but to some other ingredient in the original product, usually the fragrance ingredient. At this point, you may continue to use the new product.

If you do develop the same allergy with the new reddish cream blush, it is possible that you are allergic to the red color. Switch to a different-colored cream blush and try it for three continuous days. If you have no further problems, you may continue to use this blush.

If after switching to a different-colored cream blush, you re-develop your allergy, you are most likely allergic to one of the standard ingredients in the base of most brands of blushes. At this point, you have two choices: You can give up blushes altogether or you can consult a dermatologist about having patch testing performed to find out exactly which ingredient(s) cause your problem.

Nonirritating

Whether or not a product will actually irritate your skin—despite its claims of being nonirritating or designed for sensitive skin—is dependent upon three main factors: 1) whether your skin is normal and retains its barrier function, 2) the concentration of the potential irritants in the cosmetic, and 3) the length of time the irritant(s) remain in contact with your skin. An example is the case of a woman who applies a body lotion to her legs in the morning without any stinging or burning but complains of these things in the evening when the lotion is applied immediately after shaving. For the most part, if you have completely normal skin, you will probably have little difficulty using products labeled nonirritating or "for sensitive skin" so long as you do not leave them on for prolonged periods.

NONCOMEDOGENIC

Comedogenicity refers to the ability to stimulate the formation of whiteheads and blackheads by plugging pores. At one time, it was believed sufficient to give someone a list of ingredients known to cause comedones and to instruct him or her to avoid products containing those ingredients. Today, we know that the issue is far more complex. It is practically impossible now to find cosmetic formulations that do not contain one or more of these ingredients. Moreover, we have found that just because a product does not contain comedogenic substances, that does not guarantee that it will be noncomedogenic. It appears that many ingredients known to be comedogenic in high concentrations are not so in lower concentrations. The product as a whole must be evaluated, since it is the interaction of all the ingredients, not the action of only one ingredient, that is responsible for possibly provoking the formation of comedones.

Although a marketing claim of "noncomedogenic" suggests that the product has at least undergone some form of testing to show that it does not provoke comedones, trial and error will be the final arbiter of whether you may safely use a particular cosmetic.

NONACNEGENIC

Acnegenicity, that is, the ability of a product to provoke pimples and pustules by irritating the pores in your skin (not plugging them), is a completely separate issue from comedogenicity and is a far more common problem. Substances that are comedogenic are not necessarily acnegenic, and vice versa. As with comedogenicity, memorizing lists of ingredients known to cause acne is of little value. Whether a product causes your acne problem is related to the concentrations of any potentially acnegenic ingredients in the cosmetic and to their interaction with the other ingredients in the formulation. A cosmetic claim of nonacnegenicity, just as for comedogenicity, nonirritancy, and hypoallergenicity, should only be used as a guide for trial-and-error testing, which is the only way to ensure that any cosmetic is right for you.

OTHER TERMS

There are a number of other advertising buzzwords to be alert for. Although federal agencies exist to monitor advertisers and prevent them from making distorted, downright misleading, or phony claims, these agencies do not have enough staff to do an adequate job. As a result, you have to watch out for yourself. Whenever you read an advertisement or see or hear a commercial, you should be on your guard for certain words or phrases that advertisers love to use to hook you into buying their products. The following expressions should make you immediately skeptical: amazing, fantastic, miraculous, remarkable, exciting, instant-acting, fast-acting, revolutionary, works wonders, vanishing, and guaranteed. Scientific-sounding advertising expressions include: breakthrough, medically approved, secret formula, European or Oriental formula, amazing discovery, clinical, special technology, and secret know-how.

Expressions such as doctor-tested, dermatologist-tested, independent laboratory–tested, or allergy-tested should raise a red flag in your mind. These claims are meant to lure you into a sense of security, but what they don't tell you is who did the testing, how they did the tests, and how many tests were performed. Without this kind of information, you really have little guarantee of product value, and much cause for skepticism.

You may also find terms such as natural, organic, biological, and herbal. Often used interchangeably, these terms are meant to make you feel that the various ingredients or products referred to by them are as safe, healthy, and natural for you as sunshine and the great outdoors. There is no sound scientific evidence that shows that their inclusion in a product serves any useful function at all. Besides, the fruit, vegetable, and herbal extracts contained in cosmetics are often so heavily processed in order to prevent them from becoming rancid that they lose any natural benefits that they might actually have.

For all these reasons, *caveat emptor*—let the buyer beware—remains sound cosmetic-purchasing advice.

PART THREE

Resurfacing

6

Beauty Without Surgery: A New Age in Antiaging Creams

Five hundred years ago, Ponce de Leon searched in vain for the fountain of youth. We still haven't found it, but today, in the form of certain little tubes and jars, we may be closer to it than ever before. The end of the 1980s marked the beginning of a new age in antiaging creams, the age of the "cosmeceuticals." Some are available over the counter, and others require a doctor's prescription. The three most widely studied and most promising antiaging cosmeceutical groups to date are tretinoin, the alpha hydroxy acids, and the antioxidants; other agents that may fit the bill are 5-fluorouracil, masoprocol, and hydroquinone.

WILL CREAMS BE ENOUGH?

Fortunately, the fields of cosmetic dermatology and cosmetic surgery have undergone tremendous change in the past decade. Only a few options, such as a face-lift and eyelid surgery, used to be available for anyone wishing to improve his or her appearance; now we have a whole cosmetic skin care treatment spectrum to offer. We can now tailor-make a program for most people according to their specific needs, desires, and economic considerations.

When evaluating someone cosmetically for the first time, and before customizing any specific treatment plan of at-home or in-office therapies, many dermatologists like to classify their patients according to one of the following four skin types. (This classification of skin types is for selecting antiaging therapies, and is different from the sun-sensitivity skin types described in chapter 2 for picking sunscreens, or the skin typing system explained in chapter 3 for choosing moisturizers and cosmetics.)

Type I: No Wrinkles

Persons who have no wrinkles with their faces at rest. Usually they are in their twenties or thirties and, at most, have a few early, sun-related brownish spots visible. In general, they require no makeup or minimal coverage.

Type II: Wrinkles in Motion

Persons with wrinkles when they laugh, eat, and so on, but not when their faces are at rest. They may have the beginnings of parallel smile lines and faint roughened spots. They are usually in their mid-thirties or older and typically require some form of makeup for coverage.

Type III: Wrinkles at Rest

These individuals are usually in at least their fifties and have pronounced skin discolorations, "broken" blood vessels, and roughened keratoses (age spots). They typically require heavy foundation for coverage.

Type IV: Only Wrinkles

The sun-exposed areas of these individuals are usually sallow, gray, or leathery and consist almost entirely of lines, wrinkles, and crepiness. No normal skin is evident. They may also have many reddish, roughened premalignancies (actinic keratoses) and may have already had true malignancies removed. They are usually in their late fifties or older and have difficulty applying makeups because of caking and cracking.

Doctors find this classification system especially helpful for selecting the right therapy or combinations of therapies for their patients. For example, if you have type I or II skin, you may find that antiaging creams alone or in some combination are sufficient to keep your skin looking younger and healthier. But if you have type III skin, you are more likely to need additional skin rejuvenation methods (chapters 8 and 9). And if you are a type IV, you will certainly need them and will very likely also be a candidate for more involved cosmetic surgical procedures to redrape sagging skin, such as face-lifts and eyelid surgeries.

COSMECEUTICALS

Just when you thought life was getting simpler and that you finally understood the difference between a cosmetic and a topical medication, along comes the cosmeceutical. If a cosmetic is defined as a formulation applied to the skin to beautify it, and a topical medication one designed to alter the skin's structure and function, a cosmeceutical is a product designed to beautify the skin by altering its structure and function. In other words, a cosmeceutical is more than a cosmetic and less than a topical drug. However, there is no official legal definition for this hybrid term, and for the moment, the FDA is preventing cosmetics manufacturers from claiming that their products affect skin functioning.

What will eventually happen remains uncertain. Back in 1987, the advertising tidal wave for all kinds of supposed antiaging creams and lotions (which were, for the most part, plain moisturizers) led to an FDA crackdown on many prominent cosmetic companies. Since that time, manufacturers have been reasonably careful to advertise only the cosmetic effects of their products and not their means for achieving those effects. With the entry of cosmeceuticals into the marketplace, the beauty industry is once again going full steam ahead, and the regulatory waters are again turning muddy. For the present, anyway, as long as manufacturers don't make overt medical claims, the FDA's only concern is safety. Whether products live up to expectations is ultimately for consumers and physicians to decide.

TRETINOIN

Despite its recent attention in the media, tretinoin, a vitamin A derivative and the active ingredient in Retin-A, is not a new drug. For more than thirty years, it has been one of the premier topical medications in the treatment of acne. Belonging to a whole class of vitamin A–related chemicals known as the retinoids, tretinoin has been shown in a number of studies to have a variety of beneficial effects against sun-induced aging. Some of these effects may be seen under the microscope and others with the naked eye. Among the microscopic alterations observed after several weeks to months of daily use are an increase in collagen and elastin fiber synthesis, increased new blood vessel formation within the dermis, a restoration of a thicker, more normal-appearing epidermis, and a diminution in pigmentation (either by interfering in some way with melanin production or speeding its removal). In some cases, tretinoin has even reversed to normal certain precancerous lesions of the skin. To the naked eye, these changes show up as a rosier complexion, smoother skin, fewer brown spots, and a diminution in wrinkling. Many people regularly apply it to the exposed areas of the face, neck, upper chest, and backs of hands. In some cases, the effects have been nothing short of impressive. What tretinoin cannot do is to erase deep wrinkles and improve sagging. I generally recommend this therapy to men and women in their mid- to late thirties, when the effects of accumulated sun damage typically begin to show, although therapy may be initiated at a much earlier age if evidence of photoaging is already apparent.

Tretinoin is available by prescription only, and its application should be supervised by a dermatologist experienced in its use. Since the currently available commercial acne formulation was developed for younger, oilier, acne-prone skin, it can be irritating on drier, more mature skin. For this reason, the majority of dermatologists start by prescribing the lowest potency of tretinoin cream and work up gradually to the highest-tolerated concentration. To minimize irritation, you should apply a sparing amount of tretinoin to all the areas requiring treatment no sooner than twenty minutes after a gentle cleansing, when your skin is thoroughly dry. The concomitant use of moisturizers and gentle cleansers becomes a must in most cases. Because of a slightly increased sensitivity to sunlight, you should regularly use a sunscreen during treatment (and, of course, you should be using one anyway to prevent further damage).

Shortly following the initiation of therapy, you will usually experience a brief period of mild redness, peeling, and irritation. Thereafter, usually between four and eight weeks of nightly use, you may begin to appreciate the rosier, smoother complexion. By four months, you may see the fading of mottled discolorations, and by ten months, diminished crepiness and wrinkling. The benefits of treatment may continue to increase up to two years before peaking. Naturally, this is only a rough time frame of what might happen, since the rate of progress and the degree of benefit vary with the individual. To date, the overall experience with tretinoin has been quite gratifying. A month's supply of the medication used on the face and neck ranges from about twenty-five to thirty dollars.

When patients ask when they can stop using the medication, the answer is never. As long as the clock is still ticking and we continue to get older, continued therapy is the rule. Although some dermatologists place their patients on a twice-weekly maintenance regime after the first two years (for example, a Saturday and Sunday routine), I prefer to continue the nightly applications to ensure peak maintenance. Should you opt, for any reason, to discontinue treatment, you are likely to experience a gradual loss of improvement over a period of several months.

Tretinoin has also been used to promote more rapid wound healing after some cosmetic surgical procedures. For example, patients who began applying tretinoin two to four weeks prior to dermabrasion or chemical peels went through a significantly more rapid healing phase than those patients who had not applied the medication before these procedures. Healing was found to improve still further if tretinoin was restarted about two weeks after the surgery (the time when all the crusts are finally off and the skin is once again intact).

For all of these reasons, we anxiously await FDA approval of Renova, the emollient tretinoin facial cream specifically formulated for sun-damaged skin. This cream has been stuck in the FDA drug-review pipeline for the past several years, and it appears, according to one former president of the American Academy of Dermatology, that "approving drugs for the purposes of improving appearance is not something the agency is eager to do."

ALPHA HYDROXY ACIDS

In the antiaging arena, alpha hydroxy acids (AHAs) are one of the best-known new kids on the block. They are a group of naturally occurring, nontoxic acids that are derived from foods, plants, and fruits, including sour milk (lactic acid), sugar cane (glycolic acid), apples (malic acid), grapes (tartaric acid), and citrus fruits (citric acid). For this reason, they are often referred to in the lay press as the fruit acids. AHAs are also produced naturally as part of our normal metabolism. At present, lactic acid and, particularly, glycolic acid products dominate the alpha hydroxy antiaging cream marketplace.

Like tretinoin, alpha hydroxy acids have been around for a very long time—nearly four decades. And like tretinoin, they are FDA-approved for other purposes, most commonly as moisturizers for tough dry skin problems (e.g., Lac-Hydrin lotion) and for the dry skin associated with such problems as psoriasis, eczema, and ichthyosis, each of which affects millions of people. But their use for antiaging purposes goes back much further in time. Cleopatra was purported to have bathed in asses' milk and lemon juice (citric acid) to soften her skin, and noblewomen of ancient Rome and ladies of the prerevolutionary French court used aged wine (which contains tartaric acid) to improve their skin.

AHAs are believed to affect the surface of the skin as well as the tissue below. Research has demonstrated that they decrease the "glue" that holds the cells of the dead horny layer together on the skin surface, plump the epidermis and dermis, and restore the skin's barrier function and ability to retain moisture. Within the dermis, they may also stimulate the synthesis of the important hyaluronic acid–rich gelatinous matrix in which collagen and elastic fibers are suspended, and, to some extent, they may even stimulate new collagen synthesis. To the naked eye, these changes translate into fresher-looking, more luminous, smoother, softer skin, with fewer fine lines and less wrinkling and crepiness.

To say that the field of AHAs is burgeoning would be an understatement. Fewer than six years ago, only a handful of companies were producing these products. Now, there are more than thirty-five different companies producing more than a hundred different AHA-containing products, and retail sales of these items have reached the $350 million mark. The vast majority of these are over-the-counter (OTC) products that contain relatively low levels of AHAs, usually glycolic or lactic acids in concentrations that range from 0.5 to 8 percent. (By comparison, higher concentrations intended for in-office use by dermatologists typically range from 40 to 70 percent.) Unfortunately, not many of the manufacturers of the OTC products list AHA percentages on the label, making it more difficult to choose wisely. Nevertheless, you can at least check the ingredient list to see that the acid is listed as one of the first five ingredients, indicating that it is considered one of the active ingredients.

By keeping their acid concentrations under 5 percent, many companies are erring on the side of caution with regard to both the consumer and the FDA. In fact, the agency has received so few consumer complaints to date that it is not as yet even attempting to reclassify these products as drugs. Because some areas, such as the chest, neck, and under the eyes, are particularly sensitive to AHAs and require lower concentrations, a number of companies have produced whole AHA product lines for different areas of the body. In general, I do not agree with this concept and have had gratifying results prescribing 12 to 15 percent concentrations for patient use on all these areas. For people with oily skin, a lotion or gel formulation of AHA is preferable to a cream. Treatment may range from twenty-five to thirty dollars a month for use on the face and neck.

The timetable to see results roughly parallels that of tretinoin. Using products in the 12 to 15 percent range, you may note within about eight weeks that your skin appears smoother, healthier-looking, and somewhat less mottled in color. There may even be some thinning of roughened surface lesions. After six months to a year of continuous, daily application, you may observe diminished crepiness and less wrinkling. Peak benefits are generally realized toward the end of that time frame. Since the best maintenance schedule has not been established, I usually advise my patients to continue their daily application.

Side effects of the use of lower-concentration AHA products are minimal and usually consist of mild, transient stinging or burning that lasts no more than a minute after application. Not surprisingly, individuals with sensitive skin are the ones most likely to experience this. Irritation with AHAs is less common than with tretinoin. But should it occur, the concomitant use of moisturizers as needed and gentle cleansing routines will minimize the problem. Sun sensitivity is not a problem with AHAs—a clear advantage over tretinoin.

While the jury is still out on the antiaging value of the very low concentration OTC products, as mentioned, most researchers maintain that the relatively higher—12 to 15 percent—concentrations (some available as commercial prescription products and others specially compounded according to your doctor's prescription) are more likely to be effective. To minimize the possibility of irritation and to maximize your results, you would be wise to consult a dermatologist before using any AHA product. Of course, if you experience prolonged stinging with any product, you should also seek medical advice.

Preliminary evidence suggests that combining the daily-use AHAs with tretinoin provides additional antiaging benefits over what you might expect from either alone. One speculation is that the AHAs may in some way "re-educate" the skin so that it becomes more receptive to tretinoin. Others contend that the moisturizing effect of the AHAs may counter the irritancy of the tretinoin, making the treatment regimen more effective and more tolerable. In one proposed regimen, you apply tretinoin first and immediately afterward apply the alpha hydroxy acid (either glycolic acid or Lac-Hydrin lotion) directly over it. In an alternative plan, you apply the AHA every morning and the tretinoin at bedtime (a time when you don't have to be concerned about sun exposure). When used by themselves, AHAs are usually applied twice daily, preferably after your skin has been gently cleansed and thoroughly dried.

One final note: in case you are thinking that using fresh fruits will will give you the same effects—they don't. You can try a "toner" consisting of the juice from half a lemon diluted four to one with water, but you will not find this nearly as effective as the AHA therapies just described.

ANTIOXIDANTS

Hot on the heels of the AHAs, antioxidants are also antiaging preparations. But to appreciate their importance, you need to understand something about oxidative free radicals. Although everyone knows that oxygen is essential for human life, most people are not aware that it can also be harmful to us. As a result of our normal bodily processes or of ultraviolet light exposure, environmental pollutants, and cigarette smoke, we become exposed to highly reactive, oxygen-containing chemicals called free radicals. Although the damaging effect of these chemicals may be difficult to appreciate in terms of the body, everyday examples of their handiwork can be seen in the rusting of metal and the rapid browning of a cut apple. In our body, free radicals are the "baddies" believed to be capable of triggering cancer and biological aging.

Enter the antioxidants, the arch enemies of free radicals. An antioxidant is any substance that is capable of preventing oxidative free radical formation or curbing its destructiveness. Because antioxidants are potentially important in preventing and treating a wide variety of diseases, scientists have been actively studying these agents for some time now. Among the more well known antioxidants are vitamins A, C, E, and beta-carotene. Because investigators have found a link between high dietary intakes of these substances and a reduced risk for the development of certain diseases, it was natural to assume that in cream form, these substances might also be beneficial for the skin. There is some preliminary evidence to suggest that this may indeed be so in the case of vitamins E and C.

VITAMINS E, C, AND A

Vitamin E, or as it is sometimes also listed on cosmetic ingredient labels, alpha-tocopherol or tocopheryl acetate, has drawn quite a bit of attention over the past decade. People have been consuming large amounts of vitamin E for everything from curing cancer, revitalizing a slumping sex drive, or speeding wound healing to rejuvenating skin. Many people also continue to break open vitamin E capsules and apply the material directly to their skin to treat problems from cuts and burns to wrinkles. Others use vitamin E–containing moisturizers for the same reasons.

What we can sat at the present time is that at least in laboratory studies, vitamin E can block the sunburn reaction in laboratory animals when applied to the skin, even when applied up to eight hours after exposure. Furthermore, it is also able to decrease skin thickness and sensitivity following ultraviolet exposure. It has even been shown to have direct sunscreening properties when applied before exposure.

On the other hand, the topical use of vitamin E can cause problems. When used either in the commercial moisturization formulations or from the capsules, it is a well-recognized cause of contact allergies. I have treated a number of patients in the past several years who had developed severe allergic reactions to the vitamin E that they were applying to their skin.

Vitamin C is the most common water-soluble antioxidant in animals, and we have long known that it is essential for collagen synthesis and, thus, extremely important for wound healing. What we have learned only recently is that when it is applied to the skin in laboratory tests, vitamin C can protect against redness and damage from ultraviolet radiation. Unfortunately, homemade preparations concocted from vitamin C capsules are of little value, and may cause irritation. According to the manufacturer of C-Esta, a recently introduced stabilized cream form of the vitamin, vitamin C may also improve skin firmness, texture, wrinkles, discolorations, and other signs of photoaging after several months of continuous use. Certainly, the initial data are exciting, but more studies are needed to confirm these findings. The cost of therapy is about $35 per month for the face and neck.

The benefits of topical vitamin A or one of its other derivatives, retinol (as opposed to their relative, tretinoin), have so far been less convincing than those for either vitamins E or C. Nevertheless, this has not stopped some manufacturers from incorporating these substances into their moisturizers. All that can be said with certainty is that we need more than just the manufacturers' in-house studies to support their claims.

OTHER ANTIAGING PREPARATIONS

For many years, dermatologists have been using topically applied 5-fluorouracil creams and lotions (Efudex, Fluroplex) to treat patients who have numerous unsightly, scaly, red, sun-related precancerous lesions of the skin known as actinic (solar) keratoses, a condition affecting millions of people. The main advantage of the drug over surgical removal is its ability to find and eradicate precancerous growths even before they fully form and are seen with the naked eye. The main disadvantage—and the one that makes this therapy unappealing to many people—is that the treatment typically lasts several weeks and provokes severe redness, flaking, crusting, and even open sores within the treated areas, which last until complete healing occurs. But following therapy, many patients are delighted to find that their skin appears fresher, smoother, and less discolored. For this reason, 5-fluorouracil has recently found a place in the cosmetic treatment of photodamaged skin, either alone or, more frequently, in some regimen combining it with the use of tretinoin and/or the alpha hydroxy acids. The results so far have been quite gratifying.

Masoprocol (Actinex), a drug chemically unrelated to 5-

fluorouracil and a newcomer to the topical precancer therapy market, has proven itself as effective as 5-fluorouracil for the treatment of actinic keratoses. The redness and scaling reaction resulting from the use of this medication is generally less pronounced than that typically seen with 5-fluoruracil, and its use is therefore better tolerated. A recent pilot study by the manufacturer focusing on the treatment of photoaged skin demonstrated improvement in the cosmetic appearance of patients with mild and moderate damage after only a once-daily application of the drug for three months (using lower concentrations than those used to treat precancers). The results are encouraging, and if born out, there is little doubt that this cream will also become a regular part of our antiaging armamentarium.

Finally, one other agent that has been around for many years, hydroquinone, should also be included in the list of antiaging preparations. Unlike the other medications discussed, this substance works specifically to diminish skin pigmentation by blocking the enzyme needed to produce melanin. It is therefore valuable for lightening certain of the thinner brown (liver) spots so commonly associated with aging and for fading the dark, blemishlike discolorations that usually follow any kind of surgery to the skin.

Hydroquinone is the main ingredient in many of the currently available OTC fade creams. Unfortunately, because of their low (2 percent) concentrations, these products are seldom of much benefit. But in the 3 percent and 4 percent prescription-strength preparations, such as Melanex and Solaquine-Forte, they have proven considerably more useful. For more stubborn brown spots, however, dermatologists often have the pharmacist compound still higher concentrations, usually in the range of 5 to 8 percent. They may also combine hydroquinone with tretinoin or alpha hydroxy acids to increase their effects.

Several weeks and even several months of continuous daily or twice-daily therapy are typically required to achieve sufficient

7

Skin Freshening and Rejuvenation: Fruit Washes and Chemical Peels

Up to this point, the focus has been largely on what you can do for yourself at home to maintain healthier and younger-looking skin and to improve photodamage. Much of what has been discussed so far is well suited to people with skin type I (no wrinkles), skin type II (wrinkles in motion), and milder cases of skin type III (wrinkles at rest). But what options do you have if your problems cannot be handled by a regular regimen of adequate sun protection, appropriate moisturization, proper cleansing, suitable makeup choices, and the daily use of antiaging creams and lotions? What follows in the next several chapters is a description of in-office cosmetic procedures available from your doctor for dealing with problems that require more than home therapy. These techniques may be used alone, but to maximize their benefits, they are supplemented by the at-home methods detailed earlier. Your doctor will recommend the kind(s) of cosmetic work that can help you have better-looking skin, taking into account your skin type and your aesthetic objectives.

CHOOSING COSMETIC SURGERY

You can almost guarantee yourself disappointment with the result of any cosmetic surgery if you start off unsure about whether you really want it in the first place. Before undergoing anything, you must know yourself and understand your motivations. The decision to have cosmetic surgery has to be something you really want, and you should not agree to any procedure simply to please your spouse, lover, or some other person. Doing otherwise lays the groundwork for considerable postoperative disappointment, depression, and conflict. Most physicians, when they are aware that this kind of problem may exist, will invoke the following rule: "You earn your living by the patients you operate on, and earn your reputation by the patients you refuse to operate on." In questionable situations, they may encourage potential patients with doubtful motivations to go home, think things through carefully, and discuss their feelings openly with any other people involved. Remember, if you are uncertain why you are having surgery, no amount of actual physical improvement afterward can guarantee your satisfaction.

Maintaining realistic expectations of the outcome, no matter what your fantasies, is another important factor. Some people search for a miracle that no surgery could possibly create. You are flirting with disappointment if you mistake a cosmetic surgeon for a miracle worker capable of instantaneously turning you into a cover girl or movie star with the wave of a scalpel. Nor will disappointment be far from your doorstep if you believe that changing your appearance will automatically or necessarily win you more friends, greater respect, or a better sex life. True, looking better often means feeling better, more self-confident, and sociable, but there are no guarantees.

Less than ideal candidates for cosmetic surgery tend to be indecisive, capricious, or picky, or individuals who basically do not like themselves. They may respond to the question "What bothers you?" with, "Well, I just don't like any of it—fix it all." Or they may ask their doctors to make all the decisions for them. By contrast, ideal candidates are able to hold up a mirror to their faces and point specifically to what they wish corrected. They also do not harbor expectations that those changes will radically affect their lives.

You can avoid needless disappointment by bearing in mind the three cardinal rules of cosmetic surgery, which I always discuss with my patients:

- Rule 1: There are no guarantees. No mere mortal— physician or otherwise—can guarantee the result. What we can usually say is that the procedure is statistically successful most of the time (or we wouldn't be doing it in the first place), but that there is still a chance that improvement may be only slight.

- Rule 2: Every cosmetic surgical procedure carries with it some risk, no matter how small that risk may be. Usually this consists of the possibility of infection, discoloration, and scarring. And no reputable doctor can guarantee that complications will not occur. Remember that even if there is only a fraction of a percent risk of some complication occurring, if it should happen to you, it's 100 percent.

- Rule 3: You should expect to look worse immediately after the procedure, before eventually looking better. Oozing, crusting, and bruising are common temporary aftermaths of many procedures. Perhaps even more important, it typically takes time, often months, for certain other changes, such as swelling, discoloration, or scarring, to become less obvious or to disappear entirely. While it is understandable that you may be anxious for overnight results, you must be prepared for delayed gratification.

When judging the results of your surgery, keep in mind that your goal should be to appear no more than just your average beauty. Did you ever wonder why Paul Newman was such a female heartthrob and Christie Brinkley the focus of so many bug-eyed males? It is actually because they are average. Yes, that's right. Studies have shown that when individuals are rated on attractiveness, those with features of the norm (i.e., the average) are rated as more attractive. Using computer-digitized images of peoples' faces, researchers found that the more average the face, the more attractive it was rated. So don't vainly seek perfection from cosmetic surgery; aim for improvement.

CHOOSING THE RIGHT COSMETIC SURGEON

No doctor is right for everyone. Sometimes you have to do quite a bit of searching to find the best one for your needs. And even if you are careful about choosing, finding the right cosmetic surgeon can be quite complicated. In the past, if you wanted any kind of cosmetic work done, you went to a plastic surgeon. Today, many fields of medicine have subspecialties that are devoted to cosmetic surgery. For example, many training programs in otolaryngology (ear, nose, and throat), ophthalmology (eye), oral surgery (advanced dental surgery), and dermatology regularly include cosmetic surgery as part of their residency (post-M.D.) training programs leading to board certification. So if you are contemplating, for example, nose surgery, you could consult a plastic or otolaryngologic surgeon. If you wanted a chemical peel, you could consult a plastic surgeon or a cosmetic dermatologic surgeon.

Although a well-trained and experienced surgeon in any of these specialties is technically capable of performing the desired procedure, probably the best way to choose a surgeon is to see some of his or her work. If you know people who have had cosmetic surgery, ask them whether they were satisfied with the results and with the care and attention they received. You might also ask a trusted family physician or internist for a recommendation. These doctors frequently know the reputations, if not the work, of several local cosmetic surgeons. As a last resort, you can contact your local County Medical Society, the American Society of Cosmetic and Reconstructive Surgery, or the American Society of Dermatologic Surgery and ask for a board-certified, university-affiliated physician who performs the kind of surgery you wish.

You should select a doctor with whom you feel comfortable, and this generally means looking for one who exhibits the three As of practice: ability, affability, and availability. The decision to undergo cosmetic surgical procedures is not a small one, so you want someone who takes the time to explain what each procedure will involve and how much discomfort, if any, there is during and after the procedure, how much the procedure will cost, how much time you will be absent from work, what complications may occur, and what results you can reasonably expect. You should feel comfortable talking with the doctor and feel that you are able to communicate your concerns and fears to him or her.

A note of caution: For some time now, there has been a spate of print and electronic media advertising for large cosmetic surgery clinics, some with nationwide offices. Many offer free consultations, early appointments, and other enticements, such as same-day service, free limousine pickup, and cut-rate fees. Be very wary of any clinic that guarantees results and downplays the postoperative problems and potential risks. No one can tell you exactly how you will look after surgery, even with the most expensive computer imaging systems. Don't let yourself be talked into any cosmetic procedure you aren't really sure you want or need. And check the fees; they may not really be such bargains after all. Keep in mind that long after the surgery is done and the money spent is long since replaced, you will still have to live for the rest of your life with what stares back at you each day in the mirror.

NORMAL WOUND-HEALING

It's basic human nature—most people expect to see immediate cosmetic improvement as soon as their procedure is over and their bandages are lifted. But instead, they see raw, swollen, and oozing surgical wounds that are not attractive at all. Keeping this in mind before your surgery can spare you much grief and disappointment immediately afterward. The more you know about the ways wounds normally heal, the less you will be distressed by the process. The pattern of events and the time frames involved apply generally to wounds of all types (surgical as well as traumatic), including those from medium and deep chemical peeling and dermabrasion (see chapter 8), among other cosmetic procedures (see chapter 9).

Uncomplicated wound healing follows a fairly regular progression of stages. For about one to two weeks after surgery, the center of the wound is typically raw and oozing. Within a few days of surgery, you typically see an angry-looking reddish halo surrounding the wound edges and fanning outward into the untreated skin. Often, people are needlessly alarmed, mistaking the drainage and the reddish halo as signs of infection. Naturally, if you have any questions, or if the wound swells markedly or begins to drain a thick yellow or green pus, you should call your doctor.

Within the first two weeks following surgery, most wounds form a crust or scab. In turn, by the second or third week, the crust loosens spontaneously and falls off. At that point, the surface of the underlying skin is completely healed but usually appears intensely pink or reddish, similar in color to what you find after a scab from a scrape or cut falls off. At this point, you may safely use cover-up makeups to camouflage the remaining blemish.

During the next several weeks, the reddish color turns first to a dark brown and then proceeds to fade gradually through a series of intermediate color changes, collectively referred to as postinflammatory hyperpigmentation. After any injury to your skin, you should expect your skin to become temporarily "stained" as part of the normal healing process.

Postsurgical skin staining may take six weeks to six months to fade before your body clears the pigments responsible for the discoloration. In general, these stains fade more rapidly in light-skinned individuals who possess less overall pigment to begin with. Although the waiting period may seem interminable, it is reassuring to know that it is only temporary. Ultimately, the improved cosmetic result of the procedure generally makes the waiting worthwhile.

CHEMICAL PEELING

Chemical peels, or the application of chemicals to the skin to promote new, healthier skin formation, is a surgical procedure that requires no cutting. Although peels have been around for more than half a century, they are being used in new ways today. Dermatologists divide chemical peeling (also referred to as dermapeeling, chemexfoliation, or chemobrasion) into three basic categories: light, medium, and deep peels, depending upon the depth to which the chemical agent applied is believed to penetrate.

Light or superficial peels typically work on the horny layer and the upper epidermis to promote exfoliation (scaling, peeling). For this reason, they are ideal for freshening the skin and are commonly referred to as skin-freshening peels.

Medium-depth peels likewise affect these layers but also penetrate to the upper dermis. They work on damaged collagen and elastic fibers and are good for evening out skin tones in weathered skin and for softening or eradicating fine to moderate wrinkling, crepiness, and some forms of pock scars. Deep peels penetrate still farther, down to the mid- to lower dermis, and are therefore most suited for dealing with deeper wrinkling and scar problems. Because of their more profound effects upon the skin, moderate and deep peels are sometimes called skin-rejuvenation peels. Peels of different depths may be combined for best effect. For example, a medium-depth peel may be performed on the face, and a light peel on the neck.

There is a popular misconception that it is simply a matter of which chemical agent the doctor chooses that determines the depth of the peeling. While this is certainly an important element, many other factors also come into play, including the concentration (potency) of the chemical used (usually, the higher the concentration, the deeper the penetration) and the number of coats applied (in most cases, the more coats, the deeper the penetration). Other important factors increasing penetration include whether the skin was pretreated with tretinoin or alpha hydroxy acids (see chapter 6) or with other agents, and how vigorously the skin is degreased before the actual application of the chemical. Additionally, since different skin locations have differing thicknesses and differing sensitivities to chemical treatments, these factors also affect the depth of the peel.

SKIN FRESHENING

Glycolic acid (in concentrations of 20 to 50 percent) or trichloroacetic acid (TCA) in low concentrations (10–25 percent) are frequently chosen for skin freshening. Jessner's solution, a combination of three exfoliating agents—salicylic acid, resorcinol, and lactic acid (one of the alpha hydroxy acids)—is also commonly used for this purpose. Because freshening peels can usually be done in a matter of minutes, consumers frequently refer to them as "lunch-hour peels." The price per treatment may range from eighty-five to two hundred dollars, depending upon which chemical is used and which area is treated.

While light peels are ordinarily not powerful enough for type III or IV skin that has sustained years of sun damage, they may be quite effective in type I and type II skin for smoothing a slightly coarsened and roughened top layer of skin. They may also diminish skin dullness and sallowness; increase luminosity; lighten freckles, liver spots, and other areas of uneven or blotchy pigmentation; unclog whiteheads and blackheads; and "dry up" acne.

When performed by an experienced physician, freshening peels carry little risk of scarring, because they do not penetrate deeply. (As a rule, the dermis must be penetrated for scarring to occur.) Most people usually leave the doctor's office with only a slight, temporary (only a few hours) sunburnlike flush to their skin that is easily covered by makeup. Some flaking of the skin generally occurs in the next day or two but usually presents little problem. Skin-freshening office treatments are almost always supplemented by the regular home use of tretinoin and alpha hydroxy acid preparations.

Skin Rejuvenation

Recent evidence suggests that frequent, periodic superficial peeling, using either high concentrations of glycolic acid (50 to 70 percent) or Jessner's solution and trichloroacetic acid (TCA) in relatively low concentrations (15 to 25 percent) may in some cases yield similar results to those seen with medium-depth peels without having to weather the five- to ten-day healing time that follows the deeper peel. This form of skin rejuvenation typically consists of a closely spaced series of peels. When the chemicals are used in this fashion, you can expect an improved natural glow or radiance, an evening of irregular coloration, the softening of fine lines, some diminution in deeper lines, the softening or elimination of some scars, a mild reduction or shrinkage in pore size, and an increased smoothness.

For skin rejuvenation, I have found glycolic acid 70 percent to be particularly effective and well tolerated. In my experience, between six and twelve treatment sessions spaced at one- to four-week intervals have yielded the most consistently effective and gratifying results. A program of less frequent follow-up maintenance treatments can be individualized for each patient. Because glycolic acid is one of the fruit acids, I have coined the term *fruit washes* for its use in this series of high-potency applications for the treatment of acne and sun damage. Jessner's solution and low concentrations of TCA have also been used successfully for skin rejuvenation and usually require about four treatment sessions each before switching to a less frequent maintenance schedule consisting of periodic fruit washes. All three chemical agents may be used to treat the face as well as other sun-exposed areas such as the neck, upper chest, and backs of the hands.

Whether you have a fruit-wash series or are treated with Jessner's solution or low-potency TCA, the intent is to produce a gradual, gentler, and more controlled removal of damaged surface skin cells than you would get with more conventional medium-depth peeling. These treatments are also believed to increase gradually your skin's production of collagen and ground substance (the gelatinous matrix in which collagen fibers are suspended within the skin).

In my experience, Jessner's solution is particularly effective for improving areas that often show more severe or resistent sun damage, such as the area around the eyes, upper lip, neck, chest, and hands; low concentrations of TCA may also be used for these problems. If necessary, skin rejuvenation regimens can be customized, using one kind of chemical in one location and another for the second location.

For routine fruit washes, the prior use of topical anesthesia is seldom necessary. However, when Jessner's solution or TCA is used on facial regions, topical anesthesia may be needed to numb specific sites, especially the delicate areas under the eyes or around the mouth.

No matter which chemical or combination is used, you will probably feel mild stinging, itching, or burning shortly after the treatment begins. These sensations generally last no more than a couple of minutes before subsiding spontaneously. Water compresses are used to neutralize fruit washes and to ensure rapid relief. A hand-held fan may also be used to cool the slightly stronger burning sensations typically experienced with Jessner's solution or TCA, especially when they are applied around the eyes.

Following treatment, it ordinarily takes a few days for your skin to return completely to "normal." A faint reddish-white appearance and slight puffiness is not unusual after Jessner's or TCA applications but is uncommon after fruit washes. You may be instructed to take acetaminophen (Tylenol) and to apply ice water compresses to alleviate any discomfort, but these measures are rarely necessary.

During the initial healing period, you may experience stinging, itching, burning, tightness, and mild flaking of the topmost layer of the skin. In most instances, women may use regular make-up immediately after fruit washes and within forty-eight hours of a Jessner's or low-strength TCA application. Throughout the healing phase, it is especially important to avoid unnecessary sun exposure and to use a sunscreen on a regular basis whenever outdoors—a healthy routine under any circumstances.

MEDIUM AND DEEP PEELS

Peels performed with higher concentrations of TCA (in the range of 35 to 50 percent), or full-strength phenol (88 percent), or two-step peels that consist of first applying Jessner's solution, dry ice, or glycolic acid followed by TCA 35 percent, are the more common variations of medium-depth chemical peels. These peels have sufficient strength to improve skin color markedly and reverse signs of aging—resistant discolorations and deeper wrinkles—by causing surface "blistering" and peeling and revving up the production of new collagen and elastin fibers within the dermis. These peels may also soften shallower acne scars, eliminate thicker age spots, and eradicate some early precancerous growths. In general, the results are more dramatic than those seen following fruit washes or other milder peels, and medium peels usually require only one or two treatments as opposed to a series. Treatments typically range in price from $1,500 to $2,000.

Deep peels use a special modification of phenol solution known as the Baker-Gordon formula, and for that reason they are sometimes referred to as the Baker's peel. Penetrating as far as halfway through the dermis, deep peels offer the greatest possibility for improvement but carry the greatest risk of complications. They are useful for deep lines and wrinkles, furrows, significant pigmentation abnormalities, and thickened age spots. The typical range in price is $2,000 to $3,000.

Neither medium nor deep peeling can significantly tighten loose or sagging skin; these peels are not intended to replace facelift, brow-lift, or eye-lift procedures. Nor are they intended for removing deep or pitted scars. For such problems, punch grafting, punch elevation, scar excision, subcision (see chapter 10), buff peeling (see chapter 8), or soft-tissue fillers (see chapter 11) are much more effective, either alone or in combination with fruit washes, Jessner's solution, or low-strength TCA.

Ideal candidates for stronger peels are persons with light skin and light hair. Darker-complected individuals may also be treated but must be warned of the greater likelihood for temporary and sometimes permanent pigmentary abnormalities following treatment. In my experience, such individuals fare better with repeated applications of the milder acids, as described above.

During your initial consultation for deeper peels, a complete medical history is usually taken and an examination is conducted in order to evaluate your general health. It is especially important to inform your physician of any history of keloids, unusual scarring tendencies, extensive X-rays or radiation to the face, recent use of the potent oral anti-acne medication Accutane, or recurring cold sores, as any of these conditions can adversely affect the healing and eventual cosmetic outcome. If you have a history of recurrent herpes infections, you will likely be given the prescription antiviral medication acyclovir (Zovirax) prior to treatment to reduce the likelihood of reactivating the condition. And if you are not already using tretinoin and AHAs, you will probably be started on these, along with hydroquinone bleaching agents (see chapter 6), two to four weeks before treatment. Your doctor may also elect to test-peel a small area in a hidden part of your hairline at this time so that both of you can get a better feel for your response to treatment.

On the day of treatment, immediately prior to the procedure, you will most likely be given systemic medication(s) to relax you and topical and/or local anesthesia to numb the treatment areas. The skin is then thoroughly cleansed and degreased of all oiliness with agents such as alcohol, acetone, or the detergent Hibiclens, in order to facilitate an even penetration of the acid solutions.

In general, only one segment of your face is treated at a time, with a pause taken after the treatment of each area. The peeling solutions may be applied with gauze pads, cotton-tipped applicators, or sable brushes. Medium peels require no dressings, other than ointments. A deep Baker's peel requires the protection of a thick, masklike tape-bandage, which is generally removed after twenty-four hours.

Immediately after application of the main acid, a deep white frost appears, which will come to resemble murky gray onionskin during the next thirty minutes. Over the next several days, you will generally experience varying degrees of swelling, blistering, oozing, and crusting, which may persist for seven to fourteen days for medium peels (average ten days) and fourteen or more days for deep peels. Your doctor will instruct you as to how to cleanse the area and which topical medications to apply to promote healing. Oral acetaminophen or stronger pain medications may be needed for the first day or two after medium peels and are a must after deep peels. Once all the crusts have fallen off, your skin will most likely be bright red or pink. At this point, you may begin to apply makeup and sunscreens. The skin can remain quite red for as long as eight weeks (sometimes for more than twelve weeks) afterward.

Both medium and deep peels may result in excessive darkening or lightening of the treated skin. In general, the risk is small in fair-complected, fair-haired individuals. However, the chance of developing a temporary or permanent color change in the skin is substantially greater in darker-skinned persons and Asians. Pregnancy, a family history of brownish discoloration on the face, or the use of birth control pills may also increase the possibility of developing abnormal pigmentation.

Deep peels are far less popular among physicians than are medium peels. As I've said, although deep peels offer a more dramatic improvement, they carry the most risk. For one thing, a permanent slight loss of pigmentation is almost inevitable after deep peels (but not usually after medium peels). Moreover, there is a risk of developing a displeasing, lighter, waxy, masklike "alabaster statue" look that doesn't match the rest of the body. Phenol (but not TCA, which is nontoxic) is also known to be absorbed through the skin into the bloodstream (especially if it has been applied too quickly), and its effects have been linked to triggering severe liver, kidney, and heart-rhythm problems in people with preexisting problems in these organs. Although scar formation is a potential risk with any peeling procedure, deep peels carry the greatest risk for causing elevated scars, particularly in such areas of the face as the jawline. If scarring should occur, it can usually be treated by the application of certain anti-inflammatory creams, medicated tapes, injections, and nonadherent silicone sheet dressings (see chapter 10), with good results.

8

Dermabrasion, Buffing, and Laserbrasion

Since the beginning of recorded time, people suffering from wrinkling and facial scarring have searched for ways to improve these imperfections. Archaeological finds demonstrate that the concept of abrading skin to improve appearance is nothing new. We know, for example, that for many centuries the ancient Egyptians used abrasive pastes of alabaster and pumice particles to treat skim blemishes. Since then, we've come a long way, and today, thanks to advances in dermatologic surgery, there are a variety of safe and effective abrading procedures available to improve wrinkling and facial scarring, including conventional dermabrasion, which is still performed by some surgeons, and manual buffing and laserbrasion, which are becoming more common.

CONVENTIONAL DERMABRASION

Conventional dermabrasion is a form of abrasion, or skin planing. Used for more than fifty years for the treatment of scars—and more recently for wrinkles—conventional dermabrasion is performed with motor-driven, high-speed rotating brushes that typically operate at speeds in excess of eighteen thousand revolutions per minute.

When dermabrasion was first developed, it was mainly used to improve acne scars, pockmarks, and scars resulting from accidents or disease. Today, it is also routinely used to treat tattoos, age spots, wrinkles, frown and worry lines, as well as other types of skin lesions. Naturally, the degree of improvement varies from person to person, but most people experience somewhere between 45 and 85 percent improvement in their appearance and are quite satisfied. "Ice-pick" scars (see chapter 10) do not respond as well as the broader, more shallow, craterlike acne scars and are better treated with other methods. Dermabrasion is not particularly useful for treating congenital skin defects, some types of moles or pigmented birthmarks, and scars from burns.

The principles of abrading procedures are quite simple. In the case of wrinkles and crepiness, for example, skin contour improves and surface irregularities are obliterated when a new layer of skin, which generally has a smoother, fresher, more lustrous appearance, replaces the abraded skin. In the case of acne pockmarks, by planing down the surrounding skin, broad pockmarks can be made shallower and less craterlike. The more shallow the pockmark, the less shadowing occurs within its crater, and the less obvious it becomes.

As in the case of chemical peels, fairer-complected persons, owing to the reduced concern about postprocedure over- or underpigmentation problems, make the ideal candidates for dermabrasion. Nevertheless, many darker-skinned persons have also been successfully treated, since dermabrasion, in contrast to medium or deep chemical peels, carries less risk of causing long-term post-treatment pigmentary irregularities.

Conventional dermabrasion may be performed using one or a combination of three basic types of dermabrading cutting tools. Your doctor may choose from diamond fraises, wire brushes, and serrated wheels. These cutting tools are attached to a rapidly rotating electric drill. Wire brushes are used for deeper cutting, and diamond fraises for more superficial planing. If the pressure with which they are applied is varied, serrated wheels can provide some of the advantages of both the diamond fraise and the wire brush.

Before you are treated, your doctor should have your complete medical history and should evaluate your general health by an examination. Prior to treatment, it is especially important that you inform him or her of any history of keloids, unusual scarring tendencies, extensive X-rays or radiation to the face, recent use of the potent oral anti-acne medication Accutane, or recurring cold sores. If you have a history of herpes, you may be given Zovirax prior to the treatment to reduce the likelihood of reactivating this condition. Two to four weeks before the procedure, you may be started on a daily facial-care regimen incorporating the use of AHAs, Retin-A, and possibly hydroquinones to enhance subsequent wound healing.

Following local anesthesia, the facial skin is usually frozen solid with a skin refrigerant, such as ethyl chloride or flurethyl spray. Freezing enhances the anesthetic effect, but more important, it stiffens the skin and makes a firm surface for motor-driven dermabrasion. One area of the skin at a time is frozen and then treated. When all areas are completed, a bandage is placed over the entire face (except for the eyes, nose, and mouth). The bandage is usually removed within twenty-four hours. A full-face treatment takes about an hour.

Conventional rotary-device dermabrasion causes surprisingly little operative discomfort but is a somewhat messy procedure.

The sanding typically results in a spray mist of blood and skin. As a result, the patient must wear goggles; the staff, gowns; and the doctor, an imposing-looking welder's-like mask. Because a high-speed rotary device is used, physicians performing conventional dermabrasion must exercise extreme caution when dermabrading the delicate areas around the eyes, mouth, and nose to prevent gouging of the skin or abrading too deeply, thus triggering scar formation. Owing to this and to concerns about the possible spread of HIV and other blood-borne infections, some cosmetic surgeons have recently abandoned conventional dermabrasion in favor of buffing (see below).

For the first night or two, you are usually advised to sleep upright to reduce postoperative facial swelling. You may also be given oral medications to reduce swelling and will usually need painkillers for the first day or two. Antibacterial antibiotics may be given and Zovirax continued for several days to reduce the chances of bacterial and viral infections.

Since the first few days are marked by oozing, you should avoid alcohol consumption to prevent unnecessary blood vessel dilation and wound weeping. Within a few days, the drainage ceases and crusts form. Shedding of the crusts begins by the end of the first week and is finished after three weeks.

By ten days after dermabrasion, most people are able to return to work with the help of camouflage cosmetics. You must avoid over-exposure to the sun for at least three months after dermabrasion to avoid the development of blotchy pigmentation—particularly overpigmentation, which can result from unprotected sun exposure during this time.

Reddish, raised (hypertrophic) scars that may form weeks after the procedure are a rare (and, at one time, a dreaded) complication of dermabrasion. Nowadays, however, they can be treated quite satisfactorily in a variety of ways (see chapter 10). In certain skin types, there is also a risk of developing temporary or permanent color changes in the skin. Pregnancy, a family history of brownish discoloration on the face, or the use of birth control pills may increase the possibility of developing abnormal pigmentation.

For properly selected candidates, conventional dermabrasion in the hands of an experienced practitioner can be a useful surgical method for treating wrinkles, scars, and a variety of other surface irregularities. It can also be used to complement the results of more extensive plastic surgical procedures, such as face-lifts and eyelid lifts. The price for treatment ranges from $2,000 to $3,500.

BUFFING

Gentle skin buffing, or manual dermasanding, has enjoyed increasing popularity in the past few years. Many physicians, including myself, have abandoned conventional dermabrasion in favor of the more user- and patient-friendly buffing procedure for the treatment of a wide variety of scars, wrinkles, complexion problems (such as enlarged pores and "broken" blood vessels), and blotchy pigmentation. Buffing, which is done by hand, using sterilized abrasive material, has proven especially useful for treating the delicate skin around the eyes, nose, and lips—areas that are more difficult to treat with conventional high-speed rotary dermabrasion.

The preprocedure history and examination for buffing are identical to those for conventional dermabrasion. Because buffing is quick and easy to perform, your physician may suggest at the time of initial consultation that a small test area be treated in an inconspicuous location and evaluated a few weeks later as an aid to assessing the ultimate result of a full-face buffing procedure.

About an hour before the procedure, you may be given medications to relax you, and immediately prior to the beginning of the procedure, you may also receive a topical or local anesthesia to numb the face. After thoroughly cleansing the skin with an antiseptic cleansing agent, the doctor gently buffs, or abrades, the upper layers of skin using circular and cross-hatched motions.

Firmer pressure is applied wherever it is needed to improve deeper wrinkles and scars. In general, the many fine scratches that this method leaves at the periphery of each treatment site tend to blend evenly into the bordering normal skin, a result unlike the sharp border between treated and untreated skin that is frequently seen after the conventional motor-driven dermabrasion procedure.

In a variation of buffing, known as buff-peeling, the manual abrasion is followed by the application of a chemical agent, usually a low-strength trichloroacetic acid solution, in an effort to further enhance skin smoothing where needed.

For a few days following treatment, your skin will usually feel as though it has been overly sunburned. You are not usually required to wear a bandage afterward (as with conventional dermabrasion) and instead are simply instructed to apply some form of medicated ointment several times a day. Pain medications are generally needed for the first twenty-four hours. The time-course already outlined for weeping and crusting are much the same as for conventional dermabrasion.

Healing generally occurs within seven to ten days, after which the newly formed skin, which is typically intensely pink and slightly swollen at first, gradually develops a normal appearance. In the majority of cases, the pinkness will fade gradually within eight weeks. Regular makeup can be used as a cover-up as soon as the crusts are off, and most people are able to resume their normal occupation seven to fourteen days after either buffing or buff-peeling. Unnecessary direct and indirect sunlight is to be avoided for three to six months after the procedure, and sunscreen use on a regular basis during that time is a must whenever outdoors.

Buffing and buff-peeling, like conventional dermabrasion, cannot significantly tighten loose or sagging skin and are not intended to replace face-lift, brow-lift, or eye-lift procedures. Nor will they completely remove some types of deep or pitted scars.

For those problems, punch grafting, punch elevation, scar excision, subcision, or soft-tissue fillers may be much more effective
alternatives, either alone or in combination with buffing or buff-
peeling. On the other hand, the relative ease with which buffing
can be performed makes it an ideal procedure for quick "touch-
ups," under local anesthesia, of particularly resistant areas, often
within the convenient space of a regular follow-up visit. The price
ranges from $1,800 to $2,500 for a full-face treatment.

LASERBRASION

The word *laser* is an acronym for light amplification by stimulated emission of radiation. Simply stated, lasers are the focused
beams of certain selected wavelengths of visible light capable of
heating tissue to the point of destruction. Laser beams can cut,
seal, or vaporize skin and blood vessel tissues. For many people,
lasers conjure up futuristic images of space-age technology and
this, at least in part, may account for the mystique that surrounds
laser treatments in the minds of the general public.

Whereas not that long ago, the carbon dioxide and argon
lasers were the workhorses of laser skin surgeons, the explosion
in technology in this field has led to a whole new generation of
lasers for specific uses. At present, thirteen types of lasers are
being used, among them Q-switched ruby, copper vapor, and the
neodymium laser (Nd:YAG laser). But no single laser is currently
capable of treating all skin conditions. Because of the great
expense of many of these laser systems, they are still mainly
found at major medical centers capable of affording them rather
than in private medical offices.

Although lasers have revolutionized treatment in some fields,
such as retinal surgery in ophthalmology, they have not yet made
the same mark in dermatology. At present, the most consistently
successful dermatologic uses of lasers have been in the treatment
of port-wine stains and some types of pigmented lesions, such as

freckles and liver spots. On the other hand, claims for faster healing, less swelling, less scarring, reduced postoperative discomfort,
and better cosmetic results in treating most other skin conditions—such as warts, "broken" blood vessels, and tattoos—have
not been substantiated. In general, laser treatments have proved
no better (and often more expensive) than more conventional
therapies.

Lasers have also been used for abrading the skin, a procedure
sometimes called laserbrasion. When held a distance from the
skin, the unfocused beam emitted from the carbon dioxide laser
or, more recently, from the ultrapulse CO_2 laser, can be used to
vaporize skin tissue superficially (rather than cut into it deeply as
with a scalpel). In this fashion, the entire face may be abraded.
Pre- and postoperative care and healing time roughly parallel
that for conventional dermabrasion, and the results of laserbrasion to date have been comparable at best to that seen with the
techniques described above. Perhaps with continued improvements in laser technology and refinements in technique, lasers
in skin surgery in the future will begin to justify their cost and
the public's expectations. For now, their advantages remain
unproven. The price ranges from $5,000 to $8,000 for a full-face
laserbrasion.

COMBINING BUFFING AND
CHEMICAL PEELING

We have at long last come to a point in cosmetic surgical history
where we can customize treatments to fit the precise needs of
the individual patient. A number of cosmetic surgeons, including
myself, have found that a combination approach using both chemical peeling and buffing provides greater patient comfort and con-
venience and better cosmetic results than either procedure alone.

The combined approach targets the more aggressive buffing
for areas where it is most needed, such as the deep vertical wrin-

kles above the lip, the furrows on the sides of the mouth and chin, or for deeper acne scars, problems that are typically less responsive even to deep peels. Chemical peeling is reserved for the rest of the face, to correct minor wrinkles and discolorations. With this combined approach, the patient may conveniently and safely have the entire face treated in one session rather than two. This means needing anesthesia only once and going through a healing period only once. It is a kind of "best of both worlds" approach, and the results to date have been gratifying.

PART FOUR

Removing

9

Quick Beauty Fixes: Simple Surgery for a Younger-Looking Face

As the years pass, your face may play host to a wide variety of discolorations and growths, some with long and complicated-sounding medical names. The older you get, the more growth you are likely to have. Although most of these spots and discolorations are benign, they can become cosmetically troublesome. Doctors use the term *lesion* to refer to any lump, bump, or discoloration that in any way causes concern or differs from normal skin.

Most people seek cosmetic surgery when their growths or pigment problems can no longer be hidden by makeup. Some people, however, hold on to their unsightly growths, spots, or skin stains simply because they are unaware that anything can be done about them. Others do so because of fear: fear of pain, fear of scarring, fear of turning something harmless into cancer, or fear of the expense. Unfortunately, still others shy away because, way back when, someone advised them that "if it doesn't bother you, don't bother it." Unfortunately, many of those people confess to a profound dissatisfaction with their appearance and admit to years of attempting to get rid of their facial problems with all kinds of makeup.

New cosmetic procedures (and refinements of older ones) are relatively quick and inexpensive "beauty fixes" that can be done in the space of an office visit. These days, you can look forward to procedures that cause little or no discomfort (during or after the treatment), require little or no loss of time from work, and need minimal or no post-treatment care.

The following tells how the more common facial blemishes are best removed.

ANESTHETICS

"Will it hurt?" is often one of the first questions that people ask when contemplating any surgical procedure, no matter how minor. Because of recent improvements in anesthetics, in the answer to that question is, "very little, if at all." If needed, two kinds of anesthesia are most often used for the procedures described in this chapter: topical and local anesthesia.

TOPICAL ANESTHESIA

Topical anesthetics, or, those applied directly to the skin's surface, come in two forms: freezing sprays and creams. Ethyl chloride or flurethy spray (Frigiderm) are two freezing-spray anesthetics that your doctor may use. Because they work by temporarily freezing the surface of your skin and briefly numbing the nerves, these anesthetics are called skin refrigerants. Since their effects last only a few seconds, their use is usually restricted to those surgical procedures that can be performed very quickly. Probably their greatest use is for firming and numbing the skin prior to conventional motor-driven dermabrasion. They can also be helpful for children and very squeamish adults, for whom they are used to numb an area so that a local anesthetic may be injected more comfortably immediately afterward.

EMLA cream, a mixture of the two anesthetics lidocaine and prilocaine, has enjoyed increasing popularity since its FDA approval in the United States several years ago. The cream is applied to intact skin and covered with an occlusive dressing or plastic wrap. In order to be effective, the cream must be applied generously and must be kept on for one to two hours before surgery. The wearing of the dressing and the two-hour wait are somewhat inconvenient, but in selected patients, EMLA, whose effects may last up to forty-five minutes, can provide sufficient anesthesia to perform many different in-office procedures. Like the skin refrigerants, it is often used in especially anxious patients as a preanesthetic before a longer-acting local anesthetic is injected.

LOCAL ANESTHESIA

For many procedures, local anesthesia is needed. In this case, the doctor injects a small amount of a xylocaine (lidocaine) or procaine under the spot to be removed to numb the area. Xylocaine acts much like the novocaine that dentists frequently use, except that xylocaine works almost instantly. In fact, in most cases, by the time the needle is withdrawn, the area is already numb. Even the needle prick is hardly felt by most people, because an ultrathin needle, one much finer than an ordinary sewing needle, is generally used.

Up until a few years ago, you could expect to experience a slight burning sensation as the anesthetic was slowly injected. However, nowadays most physicians add a small amount of sodium bicarbonate (baking soda) solution to the anesthetic solution, which eliminates much of this initial burning sensation. If your doctor uses xylocaine combined with epinephrine (adrenalin), the effect of the local anesthetic will usually last about sixty to ninety minutes. If not, the anesthesia will wear off in about thirty minutes. Keep in mind that anesthetics eliminate pain but do not significantly affect the sensation of pressure. Although you will not feel pain, you may still be able to feel the doctor pressing on an anesthetized area while he or she works.

Following most in-office surgical procedures, you will usually experience little discomfort once the anesthesia has worn off. You may occasionally feel some throbbing or slight tenderness for a day or so. If your doctor anticipates that you may have more than the usual postsurgical discomfort, he or she may prescribe painkillers.

Certain areas of your face are more sensitive to the injection of local anesthetic than are others. For example, the area around your mouth, especially the upper lip or around your nose, is particularly sensitive. Your cheeks and temples are generally less so. Differences in sensitivity in various parts of your body have to do with the number of nerve endings in a particular area and with the stretchability of skin in those regions. (As a rule, the more stretchable the skin, the less resistance it puts up to the injection; thus, less pressure is required to get the anesthetic into the tissue, making the injection less uncomfortable.) For example, while most of you might cringe instinctively at the thought of a needle piercing your eyelid, this area is actually quite painless to anesthetize because it is stretchable and offers little resistance to the injection.

QUICK SURGICAL BEAUTY FIXES

SHAVE EXCISION

Shave excision is an excellent method for removing growths elevated above the skin's surface. Immediately following the administration of an anesthetic, the doctor removes the unwanted growth with a horizontal sawing motion of the scalpel blade. Shave excision essentially consists of "sculpting" the unwanted growth away from the surrounding normal skin. The resulting wound requires no sutures (stitches) and is left to heal by itself. Since the wound that is created is very superficial, there is generally little risk of scarring, and the cosmetic result is usually excellent. As a further refinement, your doctor may use the belly of the scalpel blade to scrape (dermaplane or scalpel sculpture) the edges of the wound so that they blend gently and evenly into the surrounding tissue. The usual cost is between $150 and $250.

SCISSOR EXCISION

Scissor excision, or scissor removal, is essentially a variation of the shave excision, except that instead of a scalpel, delicate, tapered surgical scissors are used to cut away the growth. Here, too, no stitches are generally required, and healing is usually cosmetically satisfactory. The cost ranges from $75 to $125.

EXCISION

When doctors use the term *excision* by itself, they frequently mean that the unwanted tissue will be more deeply removed with a scalpel and that stitches will probably be required. Typically, the surgeon cuts deeply through several layers of skin down to the fat layer. In most cases, the unwanted tissue is cut out in the shape of an ellipse, after which the wound is sutured together, resulting in a fine line.

Unfortunately, whenever skin is deeply cut, a small scar is likely to result. To make the anticipated scar less obvious and more cosmetically acceptably, the cosmetic surgeon chooses the directions of his or her cuts so that the final mark will blend almost imperceptibly with the natural tension and wrinkle lines of the skin. In addition, to prevent stitch tracts (cross-hatched scarring resulting from the use of stitches), the surgeon uses ultrafine suture material on the face and removes the stitches as soon as possible (usually no later than a week after surgery). The wound, which is not completely healed at that time, is generally redressed with thin strips of paper tape (Steri-Strips) to hold the wound edges together until healing is complete. The cost averages between $225 and $450, depending upon size and location.

CURETTAGE

Curettage is surgical skin scraping performed with an instrument called a curette, a cutting instrument available in varying sizes with a round or oval, loop-shaped cutting edge and a handle. Curettes are used to scoop out or scratch off unwanted tissue. If the growths to be removed are small, your doctor may remove them without anesthesia, since the process of anesthetizing them may be more uncomfortable than the curettage itself. Wounds from curettage are usually left to heal by themselves and require no sutures. The usual cost is between $85 and $125.

ELECTROSURGERY

There are two basic kinds of electrosurgery: electrodesiccation and electrocoagulation. Electrodesiccation is a technique that uses a high-frequency, alternating, electric current to dry up (dehydrate or desiccate) unwanted growths. The electric current passes through a fine probe that is held in contact with the growth, and the heat generated by the resistance of the tissue to the passage of the current does the job. If the surgeon wishes the destruction to be even more superficial, the probe can be held a slight distance from the growth so that only a tiny spark passes from the probe to the lesion, a variation known as electrofulguration.

Electrocoagulation and electrocautery both rely upon the use of intense heat to destroy unwanted tissue. A treatment probe is placed in contact with the growth. When the electric current is applied, intense heat is generated within the probe, and the unwanted tissue is "boiled" or, more technically put, coagulated.

Both procedures are usually reserved for destroying larger amounts of unwanted tissue, but because of that, the possibility of scar formation exists.

Local anesthesia is routinely used prior to all forms of electro-surgery, especially if large lesions or multiple sites are treated at one time. The wounds require no sutures and are left to heal by themselves. The treatment will cost between $75 and $100.

CRYOSURGERY

Cryosurgery (*cryo* means cold) is the use of freezing to destroy unwanted tissue. Destruction is due to ice crystal formation within the cells. Liquid nitrogen is currently the most frequently used of all freezing agents, although dry ice (solid carbon dioxide) and chlorodifluorimethane spray (Verruca-Freeze) are also commonly used for benign growths and skin blemishes. Liquid nitrogen freezes the lesion and lowers its temperature to –195 degrees Centigrade at its surface, and to between –70 and –125 degrees Centigrade within its core. Because of the immediate numbing effect of the extreme cold, freezing is only slightly uncomfortable, and thus no local anesthesia is generally required.

Liquid nitrogen is commonly applied either with a cotton-tipped (Q-Tip–like) applicator or by spraying. More than one application at each treatment session may be necessary. As a rule, the larger or deeper the unwanted growth, the longer the freezing time. In general, each application requires between fifteen and ninety seconds, after which the site is left to thaw. To remove some larger growths or discolorations completely, a second freeze-thaw cycle, immediately following the first, may be needed.

Cryosurgery typically produces a slight stinging or burning sensation. The discomfort peaks during thawing, about two minutes after treatment. Normally, within six hours, a blister forms at the treatment site, which in turn dries up within three days and subsequently scales off in about three weeks. The process of

freezing growths on the ears, eyelids, and around the lips is generally more uncomfortable than freezing them elsewhere on the face.
No stitches or special bandages are required for wound healing,
and cryosurgery generally poses little risk of scarring. However, since the skin's pigment cells (melanocytes) are highly sensitive to extreme cold, loss of normal skin color in treated areas
can occasionally occur. The cost ranges from $75 to $100.

COMMON FACIAL SKIN BLEMISHES AND THEIR QUICK FIXES

MOLES

A mole, or nevus (often described as a beauty mark or birth-
mark), is a benign overgrowth of pigment cells. Moles, which may
vary in color from light to dark brown, can be flat or raised, have
broad bases or grow on stalks, and can range in size from a pin-
head to several inches in diameter. Depending upon their size,
shape, and location, they may be removed by shave, scissor, or
deep excision methods.

I prefer shave excision for removing most moles, especially
those that protrude above the skin's surface. With shave excision,
the mole can be sculpted away from the underlying and surrounding skin, while preserving the general contours of the region.
However, because shave excision removes only the surface of the
mole and leaves the remainder below, regrowth or darkening of
the treatment site may occasionally occur. Should this occur, the
site can easily be touched up with light electrosurgery to correct
the problem. Those surgeons who favor deep excision of moles
point out that recurrences seldom occur with that method
because even the deepest portion of the mole is removed. But
because of the deeper cut and the need for stitches, deep excision
also poses the greatest risk for leaving a permanent linear scar and
stitch marks.

Although the sole purpose of the procedure may be cosmetic, the mole removed will most like be biopsied, that is, sent for microscopic examination, rather than just tossed out in the surgical waste bin. This is routinely done because there have been times when benign-appearing growths have been found to have evidence of malignant changes when examined under the microscope. Fortuitous discoveries of this nature have proved to be lifesaving. For this reason, while electrosurgery, cryosurgery, chemical peeling, dermabrasion, and lasers may give comparable cosmetic results, they should not be performed on moles because these methods destroy tissue beyond recognition, making it impossible for a skin pathologist to examine the mole under the microscope.

"AGE" SPOTS

Solar lentigines, often called liver spots, typically appear later in life, hence the other common term for them, *age spots*. These blemishes, which range in size from a quarter of an inch to two inches in diameter, are light or dark brown and generally appear against the backdrop of heavily sun-damaged or weatherbeaten skin. Their shape and dark coloration, resembling the liver, are probably responsible for the term *liver spot*, although they really have nothing whatsoever to do with that organ or its functions.

Lasers, specifically the Q-switched ruby, the Q-switched Nd:YAG, and the pulsed dye lasers, have been used successfully for treating lentigines and some other hyperpigmented lesions. Each of the three lasers is capable of emitting energy in a range that is selectively absorbed by melanin, the skin's main pigment, leading to its destruction and thus the fading or disappearance of the unwanted discolorations—a process known as selective photothermolysis. The main drawbacks of laser therapy are the considerable expense of the treatments ($250 to $450 per treatment) and the frequent necessity for multiple treatment sessions.

Superficial electrosurgery, cryosurgery, or localized chemical

peeling give comparably satisfactory cosmetic results in my experience. Of these, I prefer light electrofulguration, after which the
brown spots can literally be wiped away with a gauze sponge. I
find that there is more chance of prolonged postinflammatory
skin staining with liquid nitrogen cryotherapy, or trichloroacetic acid (TCA) or phenol chemical applications. An additional
advantage is that after electrosurgery, you do not need to avoid
the sun as stringently as you must after chemical applications.
The usual cost is between $85 and $125.

Solar lentigines should not be confused with freckles (ephe-
lides), which are very common, small, pale brown spots that appear
in childhood, especially in sun-exposed areas. Unlike most other
darkly pigmented spots, freckles typically become significantly
darker and more obvious after sun exposure and tend to fade in
adulthood. In general, when sunlight is avoided and appropriate
sunscreens are used, freckles cause little cosmetic concern. When
they are more numerous and cosmetically troublesome, they can
be treated effectively with lasers, chemical peels, or buffing.

"Heaped-Up" Age Spots

Technically known as seborrheic (senile) keratoses, "heaped-up"
age spots (or "passage of time" spots, as I prefer to call them) are
the most common skin growths occurring in middle to later life.
These benign, pigmented overgrowths of skin are typically thick,
"stuck-on," scaly, greasy-looking masses, which may be found in
shades of yellow or, more commonly, faint to extremely dark
brown. They commonly appear on the face. Often there is a strong
family history for their development, meaning that if you ask
around you will find other members of your family who have
them. Many people frequently mistake them for warts (see below),
which some types of seborrheic keratoses can closely resemble.

Since they are superficially located in the skin, simple curettage is by far the most effective method for removing them. They

may also be removed by electrosurgery, cryosurgery, or deep excision, although I don't ordinarily use any of these methods. Cryosurgery poses a risk of loss of normal skin color in the treated area, and electrosurgery, owing to the possibility of damage to the underlying skin by the electric current or heat, poses a small risk of scarring. Deep excision of a seborrheic keratosis, which would inevitably result in a scar, is seldom justified because of the lesion's superficial location in the skin. As a rule, these lesions are seldom biopsied; however, your doctor may opt to do so if the appearance of the growth is in any way atypical or if you have been experiencing troublesome symptoms, such as itching, tenderness, or bleeding.

"BROKEN" BLOOD VESSELS

Several different blood vessel problems may affect the face, giving it a streaked, blotchy, or ruddy look. Many people commonly refer to all these blood vessel conditions as "broken" blood vessels. In none of these cases are the blood vessels actually broken. Instead, the "broken" blood vessels are tiny dilated blood vessels (capillaries), technically known as telangiectasias. Sometimes the blood vessel that is dilated is a tiny artery called an arteriole, and because of the many "arms and legs" that seem to radiate from it, the resulting lesions are commonly referred to by doctors as spider hemangiomas, spider nevi, or spider telangiectasias.

Telangiectasias seldom disappear on their own. More often, the condition is permanent, and new blood vessels continue to appear with age. It is important to realize that "broken" blood vessels are entirely superfluous and supply neither nutrition nor oxygen to your skin. The blood vessels located more deeply within your skin are the ones responsible for those functions. All that telangiectasias do is cause you needless cosmetic embarrassment.

While the exact causes for the development of telangiectasias and spider nevi are not known, several factors seem to aggravate these conditions. Alcohol, which ordinarily dilates blood vessels, tops the list. In fact, the association between heavy alcohol intake, facial flushing, and broken vessels is so well known that many people with the condition come for treatment simply because they are tired of trying to convince others that they don't have a drinking problem.

The sun is another important factor, and broken blood vessels are commonly found on badly sun-damaged skin. They can also appear during pregnancy, although they generally disappear (but not always) several weeks after delivery. Likewise, they may be caused or worsened by constant exposure to excessive heat (the reason that so many professional chefs have them).

People who tend to be "flushers" also frequently develop broken blood vessels. Flushers are individuals who have a lifelong history of blushing easily and deeply when under emotional or physical stress or even after consuming hot beverages or very spicy foods. You might think of it this way: After years of dilating and constricting almost at the drop of a hat, the facial blood vessels eventually lose their ability to constrict normally and remain dilated and obvious thereafter.

Laser therapy, utilizing the ability of certain forms of laser light to target the red pigment in red blood cells known as hemoglobin, has been used successfully to treat facial telangiectasisas. For this purpose, the tunable dye and copper vapor lasers have most recently been used. While both these lasers represent a significant advance over the nonselective carbon dioxide laser or even the argon laser in treating telangiectasias, such treatments are often expensive, and the typical postoperative complications of crusting and scabbing do not appear to be much different in most instances from those observed with the more conventional electrosurgical methods. The cost averages between $300 and $750.

Electrodesiccation remains the most commonly used method for eliminating facial telangiectasias and spider nevi. A fine epilating needle, like the type used for electrolysis of hairs, is inserted into a branching area of a telangiectasis or directly into the central portion of the spider blood vessel. A small amount of electric current is then delivered, which permanently closes off the vessel. As the electric current is delivered, you may experience a momentary burning, stinging, or sparklike sensation. As a reflex response (not from pain), your eyes may begin to water. While local anesthesia can hinder the dermatologist by obscuring some of the finer blood vessels after it is injected, EMLA, which is applied topically, has proven quite useful in my experience for numbing the skin surface sufficiently without obscuring the tiny vessels.

Since your body is not aware of the useless nature of your broken blood vessels, your skin will often try to re-form or rechannelize (recanalize) the treated blood vessels after treatment as part of its normal reparative functions. Because of this, one or more additional treatment sessions are generally needed to achieve optimal clearing.

Electrodesiccation has an excellent track record for eliminating unwanted facial blood vessels, even in those individuals who have a dense, fishnetlike arrangement of their telangiectasias. The main complication is the occasional formation of a dimplelike, tiny pit scar at the needle placement site. In my experience, these rarely occur if the electric current is kept to the barest minimum to do the job. It will cost about $175 to $275, depending upon the extent of the problem.

A simple, but extremely effective radiosurgical method for obliterating facial and neck telangiectasias employs the Ellmen Surgitron. Emitting at 3.8 MHz, the frequency of radiowaves, these units operate at a range of little tissue alteration, and when adjusted to a very low current setting, numerous telangiectasias may be blanched in a matter of only a few minutes by lightly touching or tapping them in rapid succession. The low current and light touch required by this approach significantly reduces the risks of post-treatment pits or depressions of the skin, which are common problems with more conventional electrosurgical units.

As with the other electrosurgical techniques, more than one treatment session is usually required for optimal results, especially if there is a good deal of arborization (networking) of the blood vessels. In many cases, no topical anesthesia is required, and owing to the characteristics of the specially modified current that is delivered with the radiosurgical method, patients generally experience at most a slightly annoying sensation upon contact, which is another significant advantage over treatment with more traditional electrosurgical devices. In my own experience, the results of this technique have been gratifying and patient satisfaction extremely high. For these reasons, I prefer this method to all others. The cost averages between $175 and $275 per treatment.

Tiny Sebaceous Cysts

Technically called milia, these small sebaceous cysts closely resemble ordinary whiteheads. Occasionally, only one or two milia are seen, but more often, many may be found, especially when the skin is stretched taut. When there are only a few, your doctor may just nick the top of them with a fine scalpel or needle and express the contents. However, if they are numerous, electrodesiccation or electrofulguration is preferable, and hundreds of milia can be removed in this fashion in a matter of minutes, in most cases without anesthesia and with excellent cosmetic results. EMLA may be used topically should anesthesia be required. Following electrosurgery, small crusts form where the skin was nicked. These usually fall off within about seven days, leaving a tiny reddish spot, that typically fades within the next two weeks.

Overgrown Oil Glands

Oil gland overgrowths, called sebacous hyperplasia, are usually round and lobed-surfaced, ivory or yellowish, waxy-looking bumps. They are commonly found on the faces of middle-aged and older people. It is unusual to have just one, and several are typically present scattered over the cheeks, temples, and forehead.

Electrosurgery to flatten these growths until they are flush with the surrounding skin surface works quite well. It will cost about $85 to $100 per lesion. However, since the glands extend quite deeply below the surface, the flattened spot that remains after electrosurgery frequently retains its waxy-yellow appearance. Moreover, because residual tissue remains below the surface, the flattened oil glands tend to regrow slowly after a period of several months to years and require retreatment. At the same time, new ones often continue to form elsewhere. Cryosurgery has also been found helpful in some cases, however, the cosmetic results at best are no better than with electrosurgery, and the risk of skin color loss, as always, must be considered. Excision surgery would completely remove the growth but is not advisable because of the possibility of trading a sebaceous gland overgrowth for a line scar and stitch tracts.

VIRAL GROWTHS

Two types of viral growths commonly affect the skin: warts (veruccae) and a less well known but equally troublesome problem called molluscum contagiosum. Both conditions are not only embarrassing cosmetically but are actually infections of the skin. As such, both are potentially contagious, not only to other areas of the person's own skin, but even to other people.

Three varieties of warts can affect the face: common warts, filiform warts, and flat warts; all are caused by wart viruses, called human papilloma viruses. Common warts appear as flesh-colored, rugged-surfaced bumps stippled by pinpoint-sized, black specks. Filiform warts are soft, slender, flesh-colored or tannish fingerlike growths, which may project a quarter of an inch or more above the skin surface. Flat warts are tiny, firm, tan or flesh-colored flat-topped bumps.

For common warts, I usually use electrosurgery followed by curettage. For filiform warts, I prefer scissor excision followed by electrosurgery of the wound base. For treating numerous flat warts of the face, I recommend the use of electrosurgery alone. Cryosurgery and lasers are excellent alternatives. Because these viral infections are located superficially in the skin, scalpel excision is unwarranted for the removal of any type of wart, owing to the risk of scar formation.

Home prescription or OTC antiwart acid preparations are also sometimes recommended, especially for treating multiple warts or for use between surgical treatments. These wart therapies may occasionally be successful by themselves, but it normally takes several weeks of daily applications to achieve satisfactory results. Moreover, most people find home therapy a nuisance and often forget to follow the regimen outlined for them by their doctor. In my experience, topical therapies are most useful for treating young children, to supplement surgery, and to prevent recurrences.

Lesions of molluscum contagiosum are moundlike, flesh-colored, and waxy-looking bumps that typically have a central depression right on their peaks—shaped something like burned out volcanoes. Like warts, they are potentially spreadable to other areas of the skin as well as to other people.

While I prefer simple curettage for removing molluscum, equally satisfactory results can be obtained with liquid nitrogen cryotherapy or electrosurgery. Chemical application using trichloroacetic acid (TCA) may also be used to treat them, although repeated treatment sessions are frequently necessary. Home-use antiwart acid therapies, such as those already described, may also be helpful, although the same reservations about their effectiveness apply here. Here again, excision is not warranted because molluscum lesions are not deep.

FATTY EYELID DEPOSITS

Xanthelasmas are raised, soft, yellowish deposits of cholesterol and fat located on the lower eyelids and more frequently extending across the upper eyelids. About 25 percent of those people who develop them are found to have elevated blood cholesterol levels. That's why, before focusing on the cosmetic aspects of xanthelasmas, I routinely send all patients who have them for a blood test to check their cholesterol level.

Xanthelasmas may be effectively removed by chemical application of trichloroacetic acid (or bichloroacetic acid, a more potent and penetrating solution), electrosurgery, cryosurgery, excision, or scissor excision methods. The cosmetic results after any of these procedures is usually excellent. When treated by chemical application, larger, thicker xanthelasmas typically require several treatment sessions to achieve the desired results. The cost is between $250 and $500 per eyelid, depending upon the extent of the fatty deposits.

SKIN TAGS

Skin tags, also called acrochordons or papillomas, are small, flesh-colored or light to dark brown benign growths which usually hang on fine stalks. They are frequently found on the sides of the neck and around the eyelids (as well as other areas of the body) and range in size from a pinpoint to more than a quarter of an inch in diameter. There is usually a strong family history for developing them.

Scissor excision, cryosurgery, and electrosurgery can all be used successfully to remove skin tags. For multiple, small lesions, I prefer to use electrocautery or electrocoagulation, which generally takes only a few minutes and may be performed in many cases without local anesthesia. The resulting tiny charred crusts usually fall off in five to seven days, and complete healing occurs within two weeks. For larger growths, I prefer scissor excision under local anesthesia, followed by electrocautery of the base of the wound. The cosmetic result of both these methods are usually excellent. Cryosurgery also works well; however, I don't think the potential risk of possible pigment loss at treatment sites warrants its use. While treated lesions seldom recur, new skin tags do tend to appear with time. As a rule, groups of new tags often have to be removed every one to five years. It costs $85 to $100 to remove large tags.

10

Getting Rid of Scars

A scar is defined as a visible mark that remains after complete healing of any injury or surgical wound. In general, the more extensive the damage to the skin or the longer it takes to heal, the greater the likelihood of developing a noticeable scar. Composed of a dense accumulation of fibrous tissue, scars may lie below the skin surface (depressed scars) or protrude above it (elevated scars). Depressed scars typically make the skin seem shaded and cratered, while elevated scars cast shadows, which increase their visibility. Other factors that affect how noticeable a scar is, even if it is flush with the skin surface, are its color, size, location, and direction. For example, scars that tend to draw more attention include those that cross expression lines rather than follow them, or those that are located over the tight skin of the jawline.

Although chemical peels, dermabrasion, and filler substances (chapter 11) are used to treat skin irregularities, including various kinds of scars, some types of depressed and elevated scars do not respond well to these approaches. In such cases, a variety of other procedures and techniques may be used to correct them.

IMPROVING PITTED (ICE-PICK) SCARS

Ice-pick scars are deeply pitted, narrow scars with rigid walls, usually resulting from severe, cystic acne vulgaris. These scars get their name from their resemblance to the kind of marks that would rise from jabbing an ice pick deeply into the skin. Because they tend to pierce so deeply, however, ice-pick scars are not significantly improved by chemical peels, dermabrasion, or the injection of filler substances that are useful for correcting more superficial, less tightly bound-down scars. Three surgical methods are currently employed to remove these scars: punch excision, punch elevation, and punch grafting. Each is an in-office procedure that can be performed in just a few minutes, under local anesthesia and costs from $125 to $200 per procedure. Chicken-pox scars, which are also tightly bound down, may likewise be treated by these methods.

PUNCH EXCISION

Following the administration of local anesthesia directly beneath the scar, a cookie-cutterlike instrument called a punch, which is available in varying sizes, is used to remove a plug of scar tissue. To ensure that the entire scar is cut out, the plug of tissue removed is purposefully made slightly wider than the pit scar. Once removed, the scar plug is discarded and the edges of the wound are then stitched together with an ultrafine suture material. Three to five days later, the stitches are taken out and replaced with Steri-Strips. These are left in place for several days, until the wound is completely healed.

PUNCH ELEVATION

Once again, following the administration of local anesthesia, the plug of pitted scar tissue is punched out. This time, however, rather than being discarded, the scar plug is raised to slightly above the level of the surrounding skin and then secured by the Steri-Strips for several days until healing occurs. Once healing is complete, the surface may be dermabraded or treated electrosurgically in order to freshen up the overlying skin and to flatten the slightly elevated plug until it is level with the surrounding skin. When wider scars, such as large chicken-pox scars, are treated, the surgeon may dermabrade the surface of the plug, as well as a small amount of surrounding skin, before punching and elevating it, to further ensure a more even pigmentation following healing. He may secure the plug with a couple of stitches after elevation.

PUNCH GRAFTING

As with punch excision, in punch grafting the scar is punched out and discarded. In this case, however, rather than the wound being stitched closed, it is replaced with a snugly fitting punch graft taken—under local anesthesia—from a site usually behind the ear, a location that is an excellent match in both color and texture with facial skin. The areas behind the ear are referred to accordingly as donor sites, and the scar sites being treated, recipient sites. Once in place, the graft is either stitched to the surrounding skin or secured by Steri-Strips until healing is complete. If necessary, dermabrasion or electrosurgery are subsequently employed to level and smooth the grafts until they are flush with the skin's surface.

In many cases, even after the wounds have fully healed and all postinflammatory skin color changes have faded, a faint circular rim may be visible around each graft site upon very close inspection. Fortunately, the circular rims generally blend with the multitude of skin surface irregularities and discolorations that most people have, so they are barely noticeable unless viewed at very close distances or purposefully brought to another person's attention.

SCARABRASION

For many years, the accepted approach to scar improvement was to wait several months to a year after surgery or traumatic injury before attempting any corrective cosmetic repair, in order to allow for complete scar maturation. With the development of scarabrasion, however, this approach has radically changed.

Scarabrasion, or dermabrasion of a scar, is not a novel concept. What is new is that early buffing or dermabrasion performed between six and eight weeks after surgery or trauma—before the collagen bundles within the wound have had a chance to mature— has been shown in many cases to erase the scar. The procedure is generally performed under local anesthesia. A recent study showed that scarabrasion significantly improved all scars treated and that 50 percent of them disappeared. It also demonstrated that the six- to eight-week postsurgery (or posttrauma) treatment interval is a critical window of time; the older the scar, the less dramatic the anticipated cosmetic improvement. The cost is between $350 and $500.

For scars that are several months or even several years old, it is now recommended that the old scar tissue be excised and the freshly created wound then scarabraded six to eight weeks later. Scarabrasion has also shown itself valuable for improving the results of punch grafting, punch elevation, and punch excision. It has also been used successfully to improve chicken-pox scars and scars from shingles when performed eight weeks after the crusts have fallen off.

RUNNING "W-PLASTY"

Long scars that are in highly visible locations may be surgically camouflaged with a scar revision technique known as the running "W-plasty." The theory behind this procedure, which is performed under local anesthesia, is that the line of a long, prominent scar may be broken up surgically in such a way as to leave the scar less noticeable. This is usually accomplished by cutting out the scar in such a way so that each side of the newly created wound appears as a teethlike series of Ws. Once this is done, both sides of the wound are sutured together so that the triangular shapes of the Ws on opposing sides interlock to obliterate the wound. When fully healed, the scar line forms a jagged, "running w" shape, which ultimately results in a far less visible scar than the original unbroken scar line. It will cost between $350 and $750. For additional benefit, the resulting scar may be scarabraded six to eight weeks later.

SUBCISION

Most people are familiar with the term *excision*, which refers to a surgical procedure in which a deep cut is made through the surface of the skin, usually by a cutting instrument such as a scalpel. Because a surface cut is made, excisional procedures, no matter how well executed, generally leave a small skin scar. The term *subcision*, on the other hand, was coined because no cuts—except for a tiny needle-prick site—are made in the surface of the skin. All work is done below the skin surface, virtually eliminating the possibility of surface scarring. Depressed acne scars, chicken-pox scars, and traumatic scars usually respond well to this approach.

Prior to the procedure, the immediate area around the scar is numbed with a small amount of local anesthetic. Then a narrow needle, with a fine sharp edge, is inserted into the skin directly beneath the scar to separate the tissue and to create a small, narrow space. The procedure, which usually requires only a few minutes to perform, is particularly well suited to the office setting, and because it is performed under local anesthesia, it is entirely painless.

Immediately afterward, the surface of the skin along the length of the scar generally appears bruised and slightly swollen because of the leakage of blood and tissue fluid into the space created beneath it. The bruising is harmless and generally clears itself in two to five days. You may also see one or more tiny needle-prick marks where the anesthetic was administered and where the subcision needle entered the skin. These marks seal quickly, however, so that cover-up makeup may be applied immediately after the procedure. Some patients experience minimal tenderness at the treatment site, which usually resolves in a day or so. If needed, this tenderness can be treated with ice packs and acetaminophen (Tylenol).

Cosmetic improvement, which results from the production of the person's own new collagen to fill the space created under the scar, is best appreciated two to four weeks after subcision. It is not uncommon for one or more repeat procedures to be performed in order to maximize the cosmetic result. These procedures may be performed as early as one month later if desired. Since subcision is relatively new, it is uncertain how long the correction may be maintained. Since the skin has been encouraged to produce its own collagen, it is anticipated that the correction may persist for an extended period. The cost is between $350 and $500.

Although the risk is low, there is a small chance of developing tiny, flesh-colored or white bumps at the treatment site believed to be related to an overabundant production of collagen in response to treatment. Some areas of the face and certain individuals may be more prone to these problems. Should they occur, they can often be easily treated with excellent results in a follow-up office visit.

TREATING RAISED SCARS

There are two basic kinds of raised scars: hypertrophic ("proud flesh") scars and keloids. Both types may follow injury or surgery to the skin and at times may look quite similar.

Very firm and pinkish in color, hypertrophic scars are essentially complications of wound healing. Instead of the normal course of events in which the skin produces just the right amount of collagen and other materials to seal the wound site, in the case of hypertrophic scars, the wound-healing process seems to overshoot and produce more healing tissue than necessary. Because the excess tissue protrudes above the level of the surrounding skin, it is sometimes referred to as "proud flesh." Hypertrophic scars will often spontaneously flatten out in six to nine months.

Keloids, too, are complications of wound healing. These very firm, flesh- to ivory-colored raised scars can be similar to hypertrophic scars in outward appearance. However, unlike hypertrophic scars, they tend to grow to sizes that extend well beyond the confines of the original wound site, rather than simply being elevated directly above it.

Because of this growth, keloids can be cosmetically disfiguring. For example, when they result from ear piercing, they may hang down as large, pendulous growths from the earlobes. In general, black people are more prone to the formation of keloids, although white people are by no means exempt. A familial predisposition exists for their development. Naturally, if you are aware of such a tendency in your family, you should tell your doctor about it before you undergo any cosmetic surgical procedures.

In the past, hypertrophic scars were usually treated by "a tincture of time"—in other words, doctors usually allowed a trial of several months without treatment to see whether the scar would flatten out on its own. Today, hypertrophic scars and keloids may be successfully treated by a variety of techniques.

TOPICAL STEROIDS

For newly developing hypertrophic scars or keloids, your doctor may prescribe the application of any of several high-potency topical steroid creams or ointments, such as Ultravate, Temovate, or Diprolene. These anti-inflammatory agents are believed to work by interfering with the synthesis and laying down of collagen and fibrous tissue, thereby blocking scar formation as well as shrinking scars. They may be recommended for daily use or for use several times during the week, according to your needs.

You must be careful to apply the medication directly to the scar to prevent unnecessary thinning of the surrounding unaffected skin. Lightening of the normal pigmentation of the skin overlying the scar is a potential problem with topical steroid use, but the color usually returns to normal within a few weeks of stopping the medication.

Alternatively, your doctor may prescribe a medicated tape called Cordran tape whose sticky side has been impregnated with a topical corticosteroid called flurandrenolide. The tape is usually applied to a developing hypertrophic scar or keloid for five consecutive nights every week until the scar has flattened. Although the medication is a mid-potency (rather than high-potency) steroid, the tape serves to increase the penetration and effectiveness of the medication by locking it in. Most patients find the tape convenient to use and the results gratifying after several weeks of use.

THERAPEUTIC INJECTIONS

To ensure that the medicine gets where it is supposed to and in the highest-needed concentration, your doctor may inject a corticosteroid anti-inflammatory solution directly into the scars to shrink them. When used in this fashion, the injections are referred to as intralesional or therapeutic injections. As the designation clearly states, the steroid is injected right into the spot where it is needed. And because only small doses are needed, very little steroid actually gets absorbed into the system to cause any problems. Triamcinolone acetonide suspension is probably the most frequently used agent and is a time-honored therapy for shrinking hypertrophic scars and keloids. The cost is between $115 and $175, depending upon size, location, or the number of lesions.

Nevertheless, some may bristle at the mere thought of steroid injections. However, reservations and concerns about using intralesional (or even topical) steroids are often predicated upon misunderstanding or tales of woe from friends or relatives who have experienced complications of steroid therapy. One misconception that can be immediately dispelled is that corticosteroids have something to do with the anabolic steroids used by the bodybuilders that have caused so many problems. *They are not the same.* When complications do arise from corticosteroid use, they generally do so in patients with conditions such as rheumatoid arthritis or systemic lupus erythematosus, who require treatment with high doses, either orally or by intramuscular injection, and for long periods of time. Complications seldom occur when corticosteroids are administered in low doses by the topical method or by intralesional injection into the skin.

Intralesional injections for scars can be quite uncomfortable, since the doctor must exert significant pressure in order to force the medicine to penetrate evenly throughout the thick scar tissue. Local anesthesia may be used to lessen the discomfort. Several treatment sessions, spaced at two- to four-week intervals, are ordinarily required to flatten a hypertrophic scar. Successful therapy results in a flat, ivory-colored spot that can be easily covered with makeup. A small depression may occasionally form at the treatment site, but in most cases, this is only temporary and the skin will plump back to normal by itself within a few weeks.

Keloids can likewise be significantly shrunk by intralesional steroid injections. However, the tendency of keloids to regrow makes them generally more difficult to treat than hypertrophic scars. Laser or surgical excision, followed by intralesional corticosteroid injections or cryotherapy (the use of freezing solutions) and the application of surgical pressure dressings, are sometimes necessary to treat particularly resistant keloids.

Sometimes a dermatologist may try to soften a keloid before injecting it by freezing it with liquid nitrogen or other freezing agents and then allowing it to thaw. While freezing generally makes the injections less uncomfortable and more effective, it increases the risk that the treated area will permanently lose its normal color. For this reason, I seldom resort to this technique.

SILICONE GEL SHEETING

The use of topical silicone gel sheeting (Silastic, Sil-K, Morelle SOS Treatment) is a new and painless method for treating hypertrophic scars and keloids. Silicone sheeting is a soft, adherent, semiocclusive covering material made from medical-grade silicone polymers reinforced with polyester fabric. The treatment is simple: The patient places the material over the scar, secures it with hypoallergenic tape, and leaves it in place for a minimum of twelve hours a day for three or four months. As of yet, no one is exactly sure how the gel works, although it has been speculated that the sheeting somehow acts to decrease both fibrous tissue production and blood flow to the scar.

The topical use of silicone gel sheeting for raised scars should not be confused with either silicone injections for wrinkles and depressed scars or the use of silicone breast implants, both of which have since been banned. The sheeting merely rests upon the surface of intact skin; it is neither injected into it nor inserted under it.

Some scars do flatten completely and most show at least a moderate degree of thinning and improvement in skin color. But because the results are less dramatic than with other methods, some doctors are using the material preventively after certain types of surgery to reduce the chances of scar formation in patients who are known to be prone to hypertrophic or keloid scars. Other doctors are using it to prevent recurrences after hypertrophic scars or keloids have been treated by other means. As of now, the jury is not yet in on the precise role of silicone gel sheeting in the management of raised scars.

PART FIVE

Recontouring

11

Fill-'er Up: The Expanding World of Soft-Tissue Augmentation

FILLER SUBSTANCES

When wrinkles or scars are too deep to be adequately improved by any of the measures described, they may be substantially softened or eliminated by the use of injectable filler substances, a process known as soft-tissue augmentation. Injectable filler substances are any materials that may be injected under a scar or wrinkle to plump it up. In general, if you are able to stretch a wrinkle or scar between your fingers and flatten it, you are very likely to see improvement if a filler substance is used under it. That's why, as a rule, ice-pick acne scars, which are too bound down by fibrous tissue to improve much with stretching, do not respond well to filler substances and must be treated by the methods described in the previous chapter.

Almost everyone would agree that an ideal filler substance should: 1) be readily obtainable; 2) be easy to use; 3) be inexpensive; 4) cause no local reactions; 5) be nonallergenic; and 6) be capable of effecting a permanent correction. Unfortunately, such a substance has yet to be found. Nevertheless, the materials that are currently available or that are in the development pipeline are capable of impressive results. For now, Zyderm and Fibrel are the only two filler substances approved for soft-tissue augmentation. Additional techniques, which use the patient's own tissue for soft-tissue augmentation, include microlipoinjection, autogous collagen transfer, and Autologen.

A common misconception by the lay public is that face-lifts, brow-lifts, and eyelid surgery are the ideal procedures for eliminating furrowing and wrinkling. This notion is probably compounded by the fact that the medical term for a face-lift is rhytidectomy, which literally means a wrinkle-removing proce-dure. While it is true that some wrinkles, especially those located to the sides of the face, may be helped by the tautness resulting from the procedure, a face-lift is far more effective for removing loose, hanging skin. The rule is: lifts for sagging; fillers for wrin-kles. Don't run to have extensive plastic surgical procedures unnecessarily when you could benefit significantly, more quickly, and less expensively (and with little time lost from work) from simple soft-tissue augmentation techniques that can be per-formed during a lunch hour.

It is important not to confuse any of these substances or tech-niques with the use of injectable silicone droplets, about which there was so much negative publicity not long ago. For nearly three decades and without FDA approval, silicone, an inorganic material related to glass, was used by some practitioners in micro-droplet form for the treatment of wrinkles and scars. Before injectable collagen came on the scene, it was the only substance available for soft-tissue augmentation. However, owing to a grow-ing number of reports linking silicone droplets to complications such as the development of inflamed, permanent skin swellings (known as granulomas), migration from the injection site, and other problems related to its lack of biodegradability, the FDA has finally banned its use. Public suspicion of silicone was further compounded by the unrelated controversy over the potential dangers arising from silicone breast implants.

Unfortunately, these issues have left a lingering, unwarranted undercurrent of suspicion in the public's mind about all filler substances. It must be reemphasized that the filler materials currently available are in no way related to injectable silicone microdroplets.

ZYDERM COLLAGEN

Since its approval by the FDA in the early 1980s, injectable bovine collagen (a highly purified form of calf collagen) has become by far the most frequently used substance for soft-tissue augmentation. *Collagen replacement therapy*, the other term for this treatment, perhaps best expresses the principle behind the therapy: to replace collagen lost as a result of chronic sun damage and other aging processes.

Although newer versions await approval, bovine collagen is commercially available in three forms—Zyderm I, Zyderm II, and Zyplast—each with its own recommended uses. In general, Zyderm I and Zyderm II, which differ only in that the latter contains twice as much collagen material per unit as the former, are useful for superficial wrinkles and scars. Zyplast, which is essentially a chemically modified form of Zyderm I, is more useful for elevating deeper wrinkles and furrows. To date, more than a million people have been treated with these products. The cost per treatment ranges from $400 to $500.

Approximately 3 percent of the general population is estimated to be allergic to injectable bovine collagen. Most often, this is manifested by persistent local redness, itching, and intermittent swelling at the injection site. For this reason, two skin tests—one placed in the forearm, and the other in either the opposite forearm or hidden behind the hairline at the margin of the scalp—

usually spaced at two- to four-week intervals are routinely performed before treatment is initiated. Under ordinary circumstances, the test site, which looks something like an irritated bee
sting for the first day or so, flattens after about three days. Persistent redness or irritation for longer than this period suggests the
possibility of an allergy to the collagen itself or to any other component of the mixture. These tests will pick up approximately
two-thirds of those people who are potentially allergic.

The possible role of injectable collagen in promoting autoimmune diseases (disorders in which a person becomes allergic to
him- or herself), such as polymyositis, has been discussed on theo-
retical and legal grounds. Unfortunately, media hype over no more
than six cases allegedly connected to collagen augmentation (out
of the more than one million people who have been treated to
date) contributed to temporary public concern over this issue.
However, reputable scientific inquiry into this question has shown
no strong epidemiologic or scientific data to support the putative
link between injectable collagen and autoimmune disease. Nevertheless, persons with a known prior history of collagen vascular
diseases, such as lupus, scleroderma, polymositis, and dermato-
myositis, are not considered candidates for collagen augmentation
therapy at the present time.

The main drawback of any collagen-filler procedure is the duration of correction. In general, treated sites lose approximately 30
percent of the original correction in a matter of months, and overall, improvements may last for six months to a year, and occasionally as long as two years. It is important that you realize before
starting collagen therapy that there will be a periodic need for
touch-ups. Without further treatment, the injected collagen is subject to the same natural breakdown processes that affect all collagen
(including your own natural collagen), and the collagen is eventually cleared completely from the skin. However, subsequent treatments generally require less collagen than is needed to achieve the
initial correction.

While the need for retreatment may not seem ideal, the product's biodegradability and its lack of permanence are perhaps its greatest safety advantages. This means that anyone experiencing an allergic reaction can reasonably expect the manifestations to abate gradually as the injected collagen is biodegraded and entirely cleared from the skin.

Most physicians use the serial injection technique, which consists of delivering the collagen in a series of tiny injections extending the length of the wrinkle line. The correct amount of material must be injected for optimal results. Zyderm I, intended for superficial wrinkles and scars and containing the highest water content, is typically injected into the upper dermis. To ensure maximum cosmetic improvement, the skin above the wrinkle or scar must be raised above the skin's surface (intentionally overcorrected) to a height approximately equal to the depth of the wrinkle (or scar), so that when the water in the injectable mixture is absorbed, the skin settles back flush with the surface. During this process, which usually takes two to five days, the treated skin temporarily appears as a beadlike series of bumps resembling mosquito bites coursing the length of the wrinkle. Zyderm I, when injected through a special ultrafine needle, is also used to treat crow's-feet at the outer corners of the eyes. Because the skin is so thin and delicate in these areas, only minute quantities of material are needed for improvement, thus overcorrection is avoided.

Deeper wrinkles and furrows are best treated with Zyderm II or Zyplast (my own preference), also with the serial-injection technique. Since these products contain much less water than Zyderm I, overcorrection must be avoided; thus, treatment sites are injected with only enough material to raise the wrinkle or scar to the appropriate height. Immediately afterward, the material is molded and massaged to the desired contour. Deeper wrinkles frequently require combined therapy for best results: Zyplast to raise the wrinkle or furrow, and Zyderm I layered directly over it to soften the fine "etched" line on the surface. The results of this combination therapy have been particularly gratifying.

FIBREL

Introduced in the mid-1980s, Fibrel gelatin matrix implant is the only other FDA-approved soft-tissue filler substance for the correction of wrinkles and scars. Fibrel contains a mixture of specially treated porcine (pork) collagen and the anti–blood-clotting chemical epsilon-aminocaproic acid. Product recommendations call for mixing the material with a small amount of the patient's own blood, which is drawn, spun down, and mixed with the implant material immediately prior to treatment. Evidence suggests that the implanted material, when combined with the patient's plasma and other tissue fluids, reproduces the events that occur in normal wound repair to stimulate native collagen production. Several investigators, including myself, have used Fibrel successfully without the addition of the patient's plasma, with results equivalent to those obtained with the conventional method of preparing the product for injection.

The uses of Fibrel roughly parallel those of Zyderm I, though the method of delivery differs somewhat. For tightly bound scars, such as chicken-pox scars, a large bore needle is used to break up and loosen the underlying tissue—usually under a local anesthetic—and to create a pocket under the scar (similar to the method used in a subcision). Once the pocket is created, the viscous filler material is injected into the pocket as the needle is slowly withdrawn. Because of fluid reabsorption, treatment sites must be overcorrected, although not quite to the extent required by Zyderm I. For wrinkles, a fine needle is used, but the technique of creating a small pocket under the wrinkle and injecting while withdrawing is also utilized. The material is usually gently massaged and molded immediately after injection.

Considerable swelling and bruising often appear at the treatment sites. This is a necessary part of the wound-healing process and is believed to be needed for collagen synthesis to be stimulated. The swelling may last for about three days (occasionally up to a week) and can be eased somewhat by the use of ice packs during the first twelve hours or so.

Allergy to Fibrel has been seen in less than 2 percent of the population. Nevertheless, both the previously mentioned skin tests, although not formally mandated by the manufacturer, are recommended by many physicians before proceeding with treatment. Allergy is indicated by persisent redness and swelling at the test sites for longer than a day or two. While additional study is needed to determine the extent of possible cross-allergy between Zyderm and Fibrel, the available evidence (including experience in my own practice) suggests that the gelatin matrix implant may be a useful and safe alternative in individuals who have experienced sensitivity to collagen.

Although further studies are needed in this area, it seems that the time frame for correction for wrinkles is about the same as that seen with injectable collagen. This means that you must anticipate an ongoing, periodic need for touch-ups in order to maintain the correction. On the other hand, a large study of Fibrel in acne scar treatment demonstrated that a significant degree of correction may be maintained for as long as five years. Treatment prices range from $400 to $600.

MICROLIPOINJECTION

Microlipoinjection and its variant, autologous fat transplantation (or fat transfer surgery, as it is also known), were first used more than a hundred years ago in Germany. More recently, the technique was refined in France and brought to the United States in the mid-1980s. It is used primarily for the correction of deep facial grooves and scars and for the filling and reshaping of other profound facial contour deformities, such as sunken cheeks. It is most appropriate for areas where there is little facial movement (areas away from expression lines) and is generally not indicated for intradermal filling (filling defects in the more superficial dermis layer). In fact, filling a single wrinkle crease, even the deeper laugh lines, is rarely successful. Fat transplantation is usually performed in the physician's office.

The actual procedure is quite simple and consists of suctioning fat tissue from the abdomen or thigh through a needle and replanting it through the same needle into the face or neck to smooth out the defects being treated. Both donor and recipient sites require anesthesia. The outer thigh and abdomen are chosen because these areas tend to be the least affected by exercise or diet.

The donor site is first injected with a dilute solution of anesthetic and sterile saline (salt water) to loosen the fat before removal. The material is then withdrawn from the skin and prepared for injection. Fat for microlipoinjection may also be harvested after liposuction (fat suction) surgery (see chapter 12), at which time generous amounts of fat may be obtained. Once injected, the fat material is molded and massaged into place to prevent lumpiness. A pressure dressing is then applied to minimize blood accumulation, bruising, and excessive swelling, which must be anticipated after treatment.

Since no incisions are made into the skin, no scars ordinarily result. Instead, there are only temporary, tiny needle-puncture wounds left where the needle entered the skin, which disappear within a few days. Most patients are up and about the day of the procedure. Because fat cannot be frozen, the entire fat harvesting procedure must be repeated each time the patient is treated, until the desired correction is achieved, which may take several sessions. The duration of correction is variable, sometimes lasting only several weeks, and other times, two to three years. Because the person's own fat tissue is being transplanted, there is essentially no risk of allergy or rejection of the injected material. Thus, no prior allergy testing is required for this procedure. The cost per treatment ranges from $750 to $1,000.

Although several different filling substances may be used in the same individual, they are never mixed. However, for some people, using them in combination yields the best results. A growing number of cosmetic surgeons are using filler substances in conjunction with other modalities, such as chemical peels and dermabrasion, to get the best of both worlds. For example, using a medium-depth chemical peel combined with the use of filler substances for more resistant areas, such as the vertical, "lipstick-bleeding" lines of the upper lip, can provide the kind of significant cosmetic improvement obtained from deep peels, without the same degree of risk. Fillers may also be used as touch-ups for scars and wrinkles that persist after extensive procedures such as face-lifts, to reduce the need for repeat surgery.

AUTOLOGOUS COLLAGEN TRANSFER

Although not widely performed, autologous collagen transfer is essentially a variation of microlipoinjection. For similar reasons, it too is a technique that did not require FDA approval. In this procedure, it is not the fat tissue that is being sought for reinjection, but the fibrous tissue that is embedded within the fat. The harvested material is processed in such a way as to separate out and use the collagen-containing fibrous tissue that normally abounds within fatty tissue and buttresses it. Here the fat is discarded. The material is then reinjected into the skin, in much the same manner as Zyderm collagen. The intended uses of the material and its duration of correction roughly also parallel those of injectable collagen implants.

Because there is no chance for the development of allergies using this method, no prior skin testing is needed. On the other hand, the procedure is more complicated and requires the additional injection and resulting bruising and swelling of the donor area. Unlike the fat in microlipoinjection, the collagen prepared in this fashion may be stored for future use.

AUTOLOGEN

Another means for preparing autotransplantable collagen was developed several years ago by a company called Autogenous Technologies; once again, FDA approval was not required because no foreign materials are being injected. In this case, the collagen material is derived from the patient's dermis tissue (rather than the fat tissue) and is primarily obtained following extensive cosmetic and reconstructive procedures such as face-lifts, tummy tucks, breast reductions, brow-lifts, and eyelid surgery. The excess tissue, instead of being discarded, is shipped to the company for custom processing and storage. The technique of injection, as well as its indications for usage and duration of correction, are similar to those of injectable collagen. The main advantage is the absence of potential allergenicity. However, the difficulty in obtaining a sufficient amount of material in someone who is not undergoing extensive surgical procedures limits the general usefulness of this method.

BOTOX INJECTIONS

So far, all the materials discussed in this chapter for the treatment of wrinkles have been filler substances, materials used to plump up the depressions. By contrast, a nerve-cell–acting chemical substance produced by certain bacteria called Botox has been found useful for treating expression lines on the face—particularly the scowl lines between the eyes, the forehead "worry" lines, "crow's-feet," and the wrinkle bands around the neck—by temporarily paralyzing the tiny muscles that are responsible for the problem. Although at present not FDA-approved for this purpose, Botox has been successfully used by ophthalmologists for years with FDA approval to treat severe squints, blinks, and eye tics, and by neurologists for treating vocal cord and other neuromuscular problems.

Using a fine needle, tiny amounts of the chemical are injected directly into the small muscles under the eyebrows, which are responsible for the vertical and horizontal lines that give that angry, mad, or worried look that many people find so distressing and so difficult to control. Improvement is usually noted within two days of treatment, and maximum effect will take place within seven days. At first, treatment usually needs to be repeated every four to seven months. After several cycles, however, the interval between retreatments may stretch to as long as eighteen months.

For the therapy of wrinkles and furrows of the upper face, the medication has proven remarkably safe, with few side effects. A relatively rare occurrence is minimal drooping of the eyelid, which may last for about two weeks. Other side effects include a brief, mild headache, transient numbness in the region, and temporary bruising at the injection site.

Because of the success of this therapy in treating upper facial lines, its use is currently being studied for dealing with other muscle-movement–related wrinkling, particularly around the sides and corners of the mouth. In some instances of especially deep furrows, Botox therapy has been combined with the use of filler substances to achieve optimal correction. The cost ranges from $350 to $750 per treatment, depending upon the number of areas treated.

12

"Sucking It Out": Liposuction Surgery for a Sleeker Face

The process of suction for the surgical removal of localized unwanted or excess accumulations of fatty tissue and fatty deformities of the body was introduced in Europe in the 1970s and was originally used for removing unwanted fat from the abdomen and thighs. Following its entry on the American scene in the early 1980s, however, the technique of suction-assisted lipectomy, or liposuction (fat-suction surgery), underwent a number of significant refinements and modifications and has become one of the most commonly performed cosmetic procedures in the world. Hundreds of thousands of liposuctions have been performed to date. Its uses extend to other areas of the body, such as the hips ("riding breeches" and "saddlebags"), flanks ("love handles"), outer thighs (cellulite), inner thighs, arms, calves, and even the ankles.

Most liposuction surgery today is performed in the doctor's office or in an outpatient ambulatory setting. However, when more than one quart of fat is removed, the surgery may be performed in a hospital operating room under general anesthesia. When small amounts of fat are removed, the process is sometimes referred to as microlipoextraction—literally, the removal of small amounts of fat.

In theory, liposuction surgery is like vacuum cleaning. The cosmetic surgeon uses a thin, blunt, tubular, vacuum-cleanerlike instrument called a suction cannula. Moving the cannula to and fro in a fanlike motion to create a series of tunnels, the surgeon permanently sucks out unwanted fat from under the skin. It is believed that once this fat is removed by liposuction, regardless of any future weight gain or decrease in exercise routine, it is gone for good, and no new fat cells will be produced to replace those removed. So far this has proven true, but longer term follow-up, over many years, is needed to confirm this.

Liposuction surgery is not intended as a means of weight loss. It is not a substitute for proper dieting and adequate exercise, nor is it a procedure designed to correct obesity. To the contrary, it is a contouring procedure and is therefore generally recommended for the removal of accumulated fat in those areas of the body from which it cannot be removed by either diet or exercise. In fact, it is best suited to the individual who is no more than thirty pounds over his or her ideal weight before the surgery, and who has localized excess fatty tissue in just a few discrete areas. Although age is not as significant a factor as the person's general health, weight, and skin tautness (elasticity), the majority of patients undergoing liposuction surgery range in age from the teens through the fifties. The ideal candidate is a person in good general health with good skin elasticity.

Not all areas of the body react in the same way to liposuction. In general, areas such as the knees, hips, and ankles, which retain good elasticity, do better. Those regions where the elasticity is more of a problem, such as the "riding breeches," inner thighs, and abdomen, yield more variable results.

Liposuction of the face has been successfully used to remove unwanted fat from the cheeks and jowls and for a double chin and the neck regions, where small deposits of fat within otherwise taut skin obscure the chin and jaw lines. It has also been useful for the removal of the so-called sad pads, which are those unwanted accumulations of fatty tissue above the cheekbone and under the outer portions of the eyelid (not the bags under the eyes) that are responsible for creating a perpetual look of sadness whenever the individual is not smiling.

A short while before surgery, preoperative sedation is often given to put the patient at ease and into a semiasleep "twilight" condition. At the time of surgery, a large amount of very diluted local anesthesia is used to numb the site of the cannula insertion and the fatty tissue beneath. This important step, known as tumescent anesthesia, is one of the major advances in liposuction surgery in the last decade. The large amount of anesthetic serves to loosen the fat for easier and safer extraction and to minimize bleeding, which is especially important when large amounts of fat are being withdrawn, such as from the abdomen.

The procedure itself consists of making a half-inch incision beside the area to be treated and inserting a small tube, which is attached to a syringe or high-pressure vacuum suction. (To remove fat from the neck area, the cannula is inserted through a small incision made under the chin. To remove fat from the cheeks and jowls, the cannula is inserted through a small incision made below the earlobe.) The cannula is then swept around systematically in a criss-crossed pattern in all directions to vacuum out the unwanted fatty tissue. Care is usually taken to avoid removing too much fat, particularly when treating certain portions of the face and neck. When the suctioning is complete, the small incisions are stitched, and the resulting scar ultimately becomes almost unnoticeable. Abdomens and thighs may require thirty to sixty minutes to treat, necks about twenty minutes, and facial sites, five to ten minutes.

A growing number of cosmetic surgeons are using high-tech

computers to help them attain mirror-image matchup between one treated side and the other. The new systems give an exact second-by-second update on how much fat and blood are being removed. By knowing the precise amount taken from one side, the surgeon may suction that same amount from the opposite side. Computerized liposuction is particularly valuable for smaller jobs, such as the face, where achieving delicate, identical results is more difficult to gauge visually.

Postsurgical complications have been reported to occur in only 1 to 3 percent of cases. These include swelling, bleeding, discoloration, and the development of a dimpled or cottage-cheeselike surface appearance (more common with abdomen and thigh procedures). Tenderness, soreness, and bruising are also common and usually last one to three weeks. Blood clots, which also resolve slowly with time, may form under the skin. An elastic pressure dressing is usually left in place for one week after the procedure. For several days, the skin may feel as though it had been heavily massaged. Occasionally, there may be a feeling of numbness within the treated areas, which is usually only temporary but may persist for as long as several months. Because the incisions are small, pain and scarring are ordinarily minimal and healing is rapid. Most people are up and about immediately after surgery and can usually resume normal activities, including work, in about a week.

In general, the benefits of liposuction may first be appreciated four to six weeks after the procedure, when most of the residual swelling is gone. In the majority of cases, the results are gratifying. The cost of treating the face usually ranges from $1,500 to $3,000.

In recent years, liposuction has been combined with a variety of other cosmetic surgical procedures to enhance the aesthetic result. It is increasingly being used, for example, prior to abdominal plastic surgery (abdominoplasty), and it is now commonly performed immediately prior to face-lifts, to thin the area of fat and to facilitate the lift surgery.

PART SIX

What Else?

13

Paraprofessional Care

This chapter should not be misconstrued as a desire on my part to disparage cosmetologists, aestheticians, facialists, or beauticians. Indeed, they can play a crucial role in advising you about your options in makeup and hairstyles to enhance your appearance and your feelings about yourself. These specialists are invaluable sources of advice, for example, about the best hairstyles to camouflage hair thinning or the best ways to mask untreatable and disfiguring skin conditions. Clearly, to the person concerned by any of these problems, the advice and services of a knowledgable cosmetologist cannot be minimized.

FACIALS

Skin-care salons abound in just about every city these days, and it seems as though each has its own methods and regimens for cleaning, nourishing, toning, stimulating, and rejuvenating your skin, both during and between treatment sessions. Costs for the basic facial (which usually lasts one to two hours), when combined with the cosmetics that are usually suggested for home use, may mount up quickly. You may rightly ask: Should I be going for facials, or am I just throwing away my money? For the answer, you need to know a little more about aestheticians and what they do.

LICENSING

A lack of uniformity exists in the training and experience of professional facial-salon employees. At the present time, there are no federal requirements in order to qualify as an aesthetician (also called a facialist or cosmetologist). So far, only ten states (Connecticut, Kentucky, Michigan, Missouri, Montana, New Jersey, North Carolina, South Dakota, Virginia, and West Virginia) require a licensing exam, which may include questions on such topics as instrument sterilization and how to choose masks for different skin types. In the remaining forty states, however, anyone with a license in hair care may legally perform facials. A growing number of aestheticians throughout the United States have sought special training in clinical cosmetology. This relatively new branch of aesthetics has been working to forge a link between facialists and dermatologists, in order to deal with camouflage cosmetic techniques for burn victims, skin-graft recipients, postchemical-peel and dermabrasion patients, and others with disfiguring skin conditions such as congenital birthmarks. The trend seems promising.

CHOOSING A SALON

When selecting a salon, ask to see the licenses of both the salon and the individual facialist you plan to see, both of which, by law, must be conspicuously displayed. Look also for certificates from either the National Cosmetology Association or from Aesthetics America, which indicate that the certificate holder has passed more advanced tests and is involved in some form of continuing skin-care education training. At the same time, you should also consider the hygienic appearance of the salon: Are the floors dirty? Are the countertops disinfected regularly? Are the linens or gowns changed for each client? Do they sterilize their instruments between uses (preferably by heat autoclave), and how do they do it to prevent the spread of serious infections, such as herpes, hepatitis, and HIV? Do they change the water at least once a day in their steaming machines to prevent the buildup of molds and bacteria? You should not hesitate to go elsewhere if you do not find conditions to your satisfaction or if your questions are met with resistance.

WHAT'S IN A FACIAL

While individual salons have their own routines, most use many of the same steps. The first is usually the evaluation. For this, many facialists combine a review of a questionnaire about the skin that the client has filled out immediately beforehand with their direct observation of the person's skin, usually with the aid of a magnifier. The results can sometimes be confusing to the client. Several years ago, a correspondent for a leading New York magazine made the rounds during the course of one month to several of the largest and most famous facial salons in Manhattan. Each time that she went to a different salon, she was told that she had a completely different kind of skin. She was variously "diagnosed" by the salon experts she saw as having combination skin, oily skin, normal skin, and dry skin. The correspondent was, not surprisingly, puzzled by the conclusions that each of the facialists made about her face. A dermatologist quoted in the article that the correspondent eventually wrote concluded that "salons define normal so as to exclude most of the human race."

Aestheticians run an even greater risk of getting into trouble when they cross the boundary into diagnosing certain skin types or skin conditions. For example, there is an extremely common form of facial eczema called seborrheic dermatitis that typically causes scaling around the nose and in the eyebrow areas. To the untrained eye, this condition is frequently misdiagnosed as ordinary dry skin. As a result, oily creams, lotions, and masks are usually prescribed to treat it during and after the facial. Since the flaking from seborrheic dermatitis does not stem from dryness at all, the oily products used can frequently make the condition worse. I have treated quite a number of patients for seborrheic dermatitis that was severely aggravated by having had the wrong oily cream recommended for their supposed dry skin.

Cleansing, exfoliating, cleaning out clogged pores, and facial massage generally make up the remainder of a complete facial treatment, usually in that order. Some of the more common procedures and techniques to accomplish these ends include the use of astringents and cleansing creams, brushes, steam cleaning, facial saunas, infrared heat lamps, the use of clay or gel masks (often containing collagen or herbals), vibrators, and mechanical and manual facial massage. You may be told that these methods, ingredients, and devices are uniquely designed to deep-clean your skin, increase its blood circulation, enable your pores to breathe, tighten your pores, and restore collagen or other proteins and nutrients to your skin. But are these claims justified?

In fact, no product or device is able to get down to the bottom of your pores and clean them. Furthermore, pores do not have little muscles around them, so they cannot be exercised (or treated in any other fashion, for that matter) to tighten them permanently. And steaming can do little to get out whiteheads, pimples, or acne cysts, since these types of blemishes no longer have any pore openings to the surface to enable the trapped material within them to escape. Actually, these conditions are often worsened by steaming, precisely because the opening is closed or too small to permit the escape of any of the contents. Even blackheads, which may be more easily cleaned out after steaming, will, as a rule, reform shortly after the cleaning. If you really like the feel of it, placing a warm wet towel over your face for a few minutes will accomplish the same effects as steaming and facial saunas. Heat lamps also do little except warm your skin.

Masks, astringents, brushes, and vigorous vibrating and massaging essentially serve to irritate your skin slightly. Any type of irritation—as, for example, the kind you get by rubbing or slapping your face vigorously—results in the slight swelling of the skin that is actually responsible for that rosier, healthier look and feel that you frequently experience after a facial. The taut skin and tighter pores often seen after the facial are likewise the result of this temporary swelling of the rims of each pore (which lasts for a few hours at most).

Since nourishment comes from the blood vessels below the surface of your skin (see chapter 3), there is little benefit to the application of collagen, herbs, and vitamins, whether applied as creams, lotions, or masks.

In recent years, a growing number of facialists have added the use of electric currents and chemical-peel techniques to their regimens. So-called electro-facials, which use weak electric currents applied to the skin, have enjoyed a growing popularity for "treating" wrinkles. One kind of device that was purported to work by stimulating the underlying muscles was already declared fraudulent for cosmetic purposes in the early 1990s. You can tighten muscles all you want by any means (including repeated electric stimulation), but that won't do anything to fix the skin above.

Another device, one that is applied in the form of a gauze mask containing several electric plates, is still out there and has become a pricey and increasingly popular salon beauty treatment. Those that advocate the use of this device claim that small bursts of electric current applied to the skin's surface can restore its elasticity and rejuvenate and renew skin cells. A series of ten treatments may cost several hundred dollars. Skeptics ascribe any benefits observed from these treatments to a temporary, electrically induced irritation, which they claim most probably accounts for the observed transient smoothing (often lasting only a few hours) of the wrinkles afterward. While there doesn't seem to be any harm associated with the treatments, the jury is not yet in on whether jolts of electricity are really of any lasting value for skin aging.

Chemical peeling (see chapter 7) as part of a facial is another area for potentially serious problems. With the introduction of the alpha hydroxy acids (see chapter 6), there has been a trend among some facial salons to include a mild chemical peeling as part of the exfoliating step. Most salons are using low concentrations of either glycolic acid or trichloroacetic acid for this purpose. But peels are delicate procedures that are best performed by highly trained, experienced physicians, rather than nonprofessional practitioners who may only have minimal training. Chemical burns and scarring are potential consequences of improper use. In addition, people who are using Retin-A, in particular, may develop extreme irritation after these peels, and those with darker skin are at increased risk for developing uneven pigmentation.

After a facial, you will often find the salon salespeople pitching the cosmetics that they used during the facial treatment. They may even try to convince you that their particular "special regimen" or "complete line" of cosmetics is the only right one for your skin type. Often you are told that substitutions of any other cosmetics purchased elsewhere would diminish the benefits of the skin care program. This is clearly not so. You most certainly can substitute your own cosmetics for theirs. Even if the cosmetics you purchase from them are right for you today, your skin may change tomorrow or the next day and you could end up stuck with a lot of expensive products. If you have any problems or questions about how best to care for your skin, consult your dermatologist.

To Facial or Not To Facial

In general, I do not ordinarily recommend facials for people with problem skin conditions such as acne, psoriasis, and eczema, as the potential for making things worse is too great. Relying on facials to improve conditions like these only delays people from obtaining proper expert medical advice so that complications may be prevented. On the other hand, if you have perfectly normal skin, facials can be a relaxing and indulgent experience. In the words of one prominent aesthetician, "A facial . . . that does not give the client a feeling of luxuriant relaxation has not fulfilled its purpose." So if relaxation and pampering are what you are after, I have no serious objections to your having a facial, so long as you know why you are having it and don't fall prey to advertising hype and sales pitches.

ELECTROLYSIS

Electrolysis (also called electroepilation) is the only method designed to remove excess hair permanently. It consists of sliding a very fine epilating (hair-removing) electric needle down the length of the hair shaft until it reaches the hair root. An electric current is then applied to the root in order to destroy it permanently. Although many dermatologists perform this procedure in the office, it is most often done by a group of paraprofessionals known as electrologists.

Two methods of electrolysis are commonly employed, and many electrologists combine both methods for optimal results. One method, used less often these days, employs a galvanic current, which causes the water in your tissues to break up into electric charges and to form lye, which is toxic to the hair root. This process is correctly referred to as true electrolysis. A major drawback of galvanic electrolysis is that it is a relatively slow procedure in which only a few hairs can be treated during each treatment session. For this reason, galvanic electrolysis is used less often than the second method, thermolysis. On the other hand, the main advantage is that regrowth of hair after galvanic electrolysis occurs less often than with thermolysis.

Electrocoagulation, or thermolysis, is the more frequently used method of permanent hair removal. This procedure involves the use of a high-frequency electric current to generate tissue-destroying heat. Although electrocoagulation technically differs from true galvanic electrolysis, it is also commonly referred to as electrolysis because it too utilizes an electric current to cause hair-root destruction (lysis). The main advantage of this method is that it is faster—several hundred hairs can be treated per session. On the other hand, regrowth of individual hairs occurs about 40 percent of the time, so there is typically a greater need for subsequent retreatment with this method. The necessity of repeat treatments in order to achieve permanent hair removal is often the most frustrating aspect of undergoing electrolysis.

Although generally safe and effective, electrolysis is not without its problems and potential risks. Treatment is often painful and requires a long-term commitment. Treatment sessions may last thirty minutes each and may be required once or twice a week for several weeks, months, or, in some cases, even several years. A good result requires applying the right amount of current to do the job, but for the shortest time possible, to prevent unnecessary pain and surrounding tissue damage, which can lead to hyperpigmentation or scarring. Other problems that may arise following treatment include inflammation around hair follicles (folliculitis), infection, and acne flare-ups.

Fortunately, some of the discomfort has been minimized with the recent introduction of flexible, insulated needles that conform more easily to the shape of the follicle, slide down more easily, and reduce unnecessary tissue destruction. (EMLA topical anesthetic cream [see chapter 9], which may be prescribed by the dermatologist for use at the electrologist's office, can also be used.)

Unfortunately, as in the case of facialists, standards for the training and licensing of electrologists vary widely from state to state. Your dermatologist would be an excellent source for a referral to an experienced, and preferably licensed or certified, electrologist in your area. Examine the cleanliness of the office, and make certain that your electrologist pays careful attention to hygiene. Hepatitis and AIDS transmission are potential hazards of using contaminated needles. Don't undergo a treatment if you have an active herpes infection (cold sore or fever blister) on your lips, as the virus may be spread by contamination to other areas of your face.

Should you desire electrolysis for the removal of hairs within a mole, it would be advisable to consult a dermatologist beforehand in order to be certain that the mole is otherwise entirely normal. In fact, most electrologists that I am aware of are reluctant to remove hair from any mole unless a dermatologist has given prior consent. Since the hairs within moles tend to be thicker and more resistant to treatment, I generally perform the electrolysis on such moles myself, painlessly, with a local anesthetic. Many moles that are treated in this fashion shrink and fade somewhat after treatment.

14

Looking Ahead

The past decade has witnessed some head-spinning changes in the fields of cosmeceuticals and cosmetic surgery. I could not possibly cover all the many new and exciting innovations and techniques that are currently in the pipeline. The following, therefore, are only highlights of what I think are the more promising developments in the fields of cosmeceuticals and cosmetic surgery. Keep in mind that all the items that follow are still in experimental stages and that further testing is required to substantiate their benefits.

NEW-AGE SUN PROTECTION

Since chronic sun exposure is such an important cause of skin aging, it is hardly surprising that so much research is directed toward developing products that counter ultraviolet damage. Several formulations show great promise.

MELANIN IN MICROSPHERES

Researchers have developed a sunscreen called Prozone that contains genetically engineered (produced in the laboratory, rather than derived from natural sources) melanin. Melanin, which is responsible for the skin's natural pigmentation and for tanning, is important for blocking UVA and preventing skin cancers. A new technology has been devised in which the melanin granules are inserted into the pores of tiny microspheres or "microsponges," so that it may be easily applied in a waterproof topical form to the skin. Results in initial studies in humans indicate that the melanin sunscreen provides better UVA protection than the present commercial formulations. Because melanin cannot penetrate the skin, the cream is neither irritating nor allergenic, making it superior to available sunscreen products. Prozone is currently awaiting FDA approval.

LIVE CORALS

The clear, oozing, mucuslike substance produced by live corals may prove invaluable for sun protection. Researchers have noted that the live corals along the Great Barrier Reef near Australia are subjected to some of the highest doses of solar radiation anywhere in the world, and they not only survive in it, they thrive in it. Australian researchers have synthesized and patented what they think is the chemical responsible for this protection and are currently working on incorporating it into commercial sunscreen preparations and cosmetics to improve the UV protective benefits. More research is needed to confirm these findings.

TOPICAL VITAMIN C

Topical vitamin C, already discussed for its antioxidant properties, may well prove useful for preventing sun-baked skin from wrinkling and developing skin cancers. After application of a lotion formulation that is being tested—containing about a 10 percent concentration (about 20 times 'its normal concentration in the skin)—the vitamin C is believed to bind to the skin within minutes and cannot be washed off. The vitamin C is believed to function not as a sunscreen but by interfering with the chemical reaction that actually causes damage when the ultraviolet light hits the skin. Because of a reservoir effect within the skin, it is believed to work for a period of up to three days after a single application. Vitamin C protects against the development of sunburn, and because of its anti-inflammatory effects, it may also be useful for treating sunburn. The results of ongoing testing are eagerly awaited.

DNA Fragments and Tanning

Significant inroads have also been made in our understanding of the tanning process. Investigators have discovered that tanning, which has been characterized as an SOS response of the skin to UV light, is ordinarily not triggered until DNA damage is produced by sunlight and repair of the damage has begun. To reproduce the tanning process safely, researchers spread a simple DNA fragment made in the laboratory onto the skin of laboratory animals, and they were able to trigger a natural, protective tan without provoking any damage to the skin. In contrast, existing sunless tanning lotions merely stain the skin and offer no protection because they do not stimulate melanin production. These exciting preliminary findings await confirmation by human testing.

DNA Repair

Since direct ultraviolet damage to the genetic material of skin cells is believed responsible for so much of the medical and cosmetic damage to our skin, anything that can reverse that damage would be welcomed. For now, an enzyme capable of DNA-repair, produced by genetically engineered bacteria and known as T4N5, may do just that. Test-tube studies have shown enhancement of ultraviolet repair of the cellular genetic code when this enzyme is present, suggesting that a topical preparation of this enzyme could be useful for reversing sun-damaged skin. If this proves so in tests in humans, it will be the first preparation capable of reversing sun-induced genetic damage *after* exposure.

PREVENTING SCARS

Despite all the wonders of cosmetic surgery, the problem of scarring still exists. Perhaps one of the most promising—and possibly revolutionary—discoveries in scar prevention and therapy relates to the growth factor known as TGF beta (transformation growth factor beta). Growth factors are substances that regulate the growth and development of cells and play a critical role in many body functions. Hundreds of these chemicals have been identified in the past few years, and their individual functions are now beginning to be understood. Biologists investigating why fetuses' wounds heal without the inflammation and scarring that plagues all of us after birth discovered that TGF beta was strangely absent in fetal wounds, as compared to normal wounds.

Reasoning that the TGF beta may have been used up in some way by the process of fetal wound healing and therefore was the most likely candidate responsible for the remarkable healing observed, the biologists tried injecting and swabbing the growth factor into the sides of surgical wounds in adults and found that scar formation stopped. If the findings from this study are born out in larger trials, the material will no doubt find future use with burn and trauma victims. The treatment has the added advantages of being relatively inexpensive, demanding little technology to produce the material, and requiring minimal expertise to administer it. For now, we must await the results of further testing with cautious optimism.

NEW WRINKLE FIGHTERS

GORE-TEX

A somewhat novel approach to wrinkle correction—the use of Gore-Tex suture, a nonabsorbable monofilament suture material—is being tested by European investigators. The material, an expanded polytetrafluoretheylene suture material, has been safely used for years by surgeons for wound repair: Using a long straight needle, the suture is threaded back and forth through the deep dermis directly under each wrinkle as many times as needed to achieve the desired correction, and then trimmed. Because the suture material is left in place under the skin and is not broken down by the body, the results of this technique are not only immediate but permanent. Of those treated in this fashion, 10 percent have experienced a minor irritation along the track of the suture, which cleared in one to two days. To date, the material has not provoked any true allergic reactions. More research is needed, however, to define the role of this material in correcting wrinkles.

ELECTRORYDESIS

Electrorydesis is the use of an electromagnetic field introduced superficially into the skin by microneedles to correct wrinkles. The idea is based on experimental findings in the laboratory that the use of a pulsed electromagnetic field can increase the production of DNA, collagen, and hyaluronic acid. Initial studies in human volunteers, following a series of six weekly treatments, showed significant softening of wrinkles. The duration of the correction is still being studied, and more research is needed to understand the role of electromagnetic fields in tissue repair.

HYLAN GEL

Highly encouraging preliminary evaluations of a new biomaterial known as hylan gel suggest that it may play a significant role in soft-tissue augmentation. Hylan is a derivative of hyaluronic acid, the primary component of the gelatinous ground substance within the dermis that supports the collagen and elastin fibers. Hyaluronic acid medical products have been around since the early 1980s and have already been successfully used in fields such as ophthalmology. The unique properties of the hylan material (which may be extracted from natural sources or bioengineered in the laboratory) and its impressive safety profile as a filler substance to date in human trials are extremely encouraging. The material has not yet provoked any allergic reactions, so skin testing, unlike with collagen and gelatin-matrix materials, is not required. In addition, although the method of injecting the gel is similar to that used for collagen, hylan can be placed into both superficial and deep locations in a single treatment session and massaged and molded into place. No significant complications of any kind have been noted in initial studies, and the wrinkle corrections have been observed to last longer than those performed with collagen. FDA approval for this material, which has been actively tested since early 1991, is eagerly awaited.

A FINAL REFLECTION

If the last decade is any indication of our rate of progress in the realm of holding back the hands of time, the next decade carrying us into the new millennium clearly holds promise for some of the most exciting possibilities for looking better and younger. We can reasonably anticipate seeing antiaging creams and lotions that penetrate more efficiently and more rapidly and produce dramatic softening and elimination of lines and wrinkles. We can expect better, more versatile, and longer-lasting filler substances, and we will no doubt see the development of improved, virtually painless procedures for quickly eliminating everything from broken blood vessels to detracting lumps, bumps, and marks in the space of a coffee break. The current trend suggests that the next few years are going to be a great time for looking great.

Index